SOAP MAKING RECIPES

The Complete Know How Book to Soap Making

(Soap Making Book With Simple and Gentle Soap Recipes for Sensitive Skin)

Jack Weeks

Published by Oliver Leish

Jack Weeks

All Rights Reserved

Soap Making Recipes: The Complete Know How Book to Soap Making (Soap Making Book With Simple and Gentle Soap Recipes for Sensitive Skin)

ISBN 978-1-77485-080-0

All rights reserved. No part of this guide may be reproduced in any form without permission in writing from the publisher except in the case of brief quotations embodied in critical articles or reviews.

Legal & Disclaimer

The information contained in this book is not designed to replace or take the place of any form of medicine or professional medical advice. The information in this book has been provided for educational and entertainment purposes only.

The information contained in this book has been compiled from sources deemed reliable, and it is accurate to the best of the Author's knowledge; however, the Author cannot guarantee its accuracy and validity and cannot be held liable for any errors or omissions. Changes are periodically made to this book. You must consult your doctor or get professional medical advice before using any of the suggested remedies, techniques, or information in this book.

Upon using the information contained in this book, you agree to hold harmless the Author from and against any damages, costs, and expenses, including any legal fees potentially resulting from the application of any of the information provided by this guide. This disclaimer applies to any damages or injury caused by the use and application, whether directly or indirectly, of any advice or information presented, whether for breach of contract, tort, negligence, personal injury, criminal intent, or under any other cause of action.

You agree to accept all risks of using the information presented inside this book. You need to consult a professional medical practitioner in order to ensure you are both able and healthy enough to participate in this program.

Table of Contents

INTRODUCTION 1

CHAPTER 1: THE ART OF SOAP CRAFTING 4

CHAPTER 2: THE SQUEAKY CLEAN TRUTH ABOUT SOAPS .. 9

CHAPTER 3: SIMPLE SOAP RECIPES 28

MELT-AND-POUR SOAP RECIPES 28

    APPLE PIE SOAP 28

    BLACK RASPBERRY SOAP 30

    CINNAMON SOAP 31

    CRANBERRY VANILLA SOAP 33

    EARL GREY TEA SOAP 34

    FLOWER CUPCAKE SOAP.. 36

    GINGERBREAD SOAP 37

    GOAT'S MILK LEMON SOAP 39

    GRAPEFRUIT SOAP WITH HIMALAYAN SALT 40

    HONEY AND OATMEAL SOAP 42

    HONEYSUCKLE SOAP 43

    LEMON POPPY SEED SOAP 45

    LIME AND CILANTRO SOAP 46

    LEMON AND RASPBERRY SOAP 47

    LEMONGRASS SOAP 49

Milk And Honey Soap 50

Orange And Bergamot Soap 52

Orange Turmeric Soap.. 53

Patchouli Charcoal Soap... 55

Pumpkin Spice Soap... 56

Rose Loofah Soap 57

Spiced Apple Soap 59

Sweet Almond Soap... 60

Vanilla Latte Soap... 61

White Tea And Ginger Loofah Soap 63

COLD-PROCESS SOAP RECIPES 65

Castile Soap 65

Coconut Soap 66

Lard Soap 68

Basic Tallow Soap 70

Tallow Soap With Honey 72

Basic Cold-Process Soap 73

Basic Vegan Soap 75

Bastille Soap.. 77

Supermarket Soap 79

Supermarket Soap With Shea Butter.................................. 81

Lavender Soap 83

CHAPTER 4: EQUIPMENT AND SUPPLIES REQUIRED 85

CHAPTER 5: NATURAL SOAP MAKING 91

CHAPTER 6: STEP BY STEP SOAP MAKING PROCESS 104

CHAPTER 7: SOAP RECIPES YOU CAN MAKE AT HOME .. 116

OATMEAL CINNAMON EXFOLIATING BAR 116

LEMON CHIA MOISTURIZING SCRUB SOAP 117

VANILLA ROSE MOISTURIZING SOAP 119

SWEET STRAWBERRY SOAP 121

FULL DETOX ANTI ACNE BAR 123

COCONUT MILK MOISTURIZING SOAP 125

ACTIVATED CHARCOAL SOAP 127

SKIN BRIGHTENING ANTI-AGING SOAP 129

ROSEMARY COOLING SOAP 130

LAZY SUMMER DAY SOOTHING SOAP 131

ENGLISH GARDEN CLEANSING BAR 133

MORNING COFFEE EXFOLIATING BAR 135

CHOCOLATE MINT EXFOLIATING BAR 136

LAVENDER FIELDS MOISTURIZING SOAP 138

OASIS DREAMS MOISTURIZING SOAP 140

FLORAL CLEAR SKIN SOAP 141

COOL AND REFRESHING ANTI SPOT SOAP 144

ALMOND MILK ANTI-AGING SOAP 145

LA VIE EN ROSE NOURISHING BAR 146

SPRING BLOOMS NOURISHING BAR 148

CHAPTER 8: SOAP-MAKING METHODS 150

CHAPTER 9: HOT PROCESSED SOAPS 155

Coffee Antioxidant Soap 155

Avocado And Mango Swirl Soap 157

CHAPTER 10: HOMEMADE SOAP FOR EXFOLIATION 161

CHAPTER 11: EASY TECHNIQUES FOR NEWBIES 171

CHAPTER 12: HOT PROCESS SOAP MAKING 176

CONCLUSION 190

Introduction

As someone who is passionate about life and is also creative, I am always looking for new ways to make my life more beautiful and healthier. That being said, a few years ago, I've stumbled upon a handmade soap recipe and decided to give it a try. At first, the process of soap making seemed so confusing to me, but with time and practice, I learned how to do it the best way.

Now, you must be thinking: "Why would I waste time on making soap bars when I can just go to the store and buy them"? Well, of course, you can, but do you really want to? Stop for a second and think about all the ingredients that a manufacturer puts into the soap bar. Do you know which ingredients they use? That's how I thought – you have no idea of how harmful that soap may be to your skin.

So, tell me, would not be much smarter to buy all of the ingredients and invest some time in making your very own soap? If you are anything like me, then you take care of your skin and the way you treat it. Handmade soap bars are great for cleaning and hydrating your skin. Add to that your favorite color or scent and you turned a bath time into a sensational ritual.

The best part of making homemade soap bars is that you get to choose what ingredients you will put in the mixture. This is especially great if you have a sensitive skin since you can add the ingredients that will soothe it and make it softer. One more thing I love about soap making is fun. Once you learn how to make soap bars, you will have so much fun every time you want to make soap bars, because possibilities are endless. Soap making will be as creative and fun as you are, so don't be afraid to set free your creativity and embrace fresh ideas. Speaking of which, in this e-book, I want to share 50 great homemade soap recipes, so as to boost your creativity. Thanks to these recipes, you will forget about commercial soap bars once and for all.

Chapter 1: The Art Of Soap Crafting

And Why You Should Whip Up Your Own Soap

Common lore about how soaps were initially discovered states that the ashes from sacrifices mingled with the fat left after these sacrifices and washed into the river, creating a foam. People then discovered that this foam was actually a very cleansing one and soap crafting grew from there.

And yes, it really can be that simple. All you need to is mix a fat, such as tallow, with an alkaline. In pioneer days, soap was a very practical homemade affair mixing the wood ash from fires with rendered fat and drippings.

Nowadays, we use caustic soda in place of wood ash and this does give people a little cause for concern as it can burn the skin if incorrectly used. That said, as long as you follow the safety protocols that I have laid out in this book, you can easily and safely use the lye.

At this point, you may be wondering whether or not it is even worthwhile to make soaps from scratch. After all, isn't it so much simpler to pick up a bar at the department store? I cannot fault that logic, it is far simpler to get a bar at a department store but, in truth you are not getting soap at all. What you are getting is a bunch of synthetic chemicals designed to create a good lather (because consumers expect the lather). These "soaps" will clean your skin but they are very drying and you can never be completely sure what is put into them.

That is why we are told today that we should never wash our faces with soap – it is too drying for the delicate facial skin. When you use natural, real soap, however, you do not need to worry about damaging the acid mantle of the skin or drying the skin out excessively.

I, and everyone in my family use soap to wash our faces with – real soap that we have made ourselves. The big plus when it comes to making your own soap is that you can custom make it to fit your actual skin conditions.

Eczema is something that plagues everyone in our family from time to time and, at one stage, I was simply unable to get rid of it. I consulted doctors and dermatologists but was never able to clear it up completely. That is actually one of the reasons that I started looking into making my own soaps and body lotions.

I have not looked back since. The eczema will flare up once in a while when I am under a lot of stress but, by and large, I consider it gone. When I do have attacks now, they are not nearly as bad and last for a much shorter duration.

Whether you have eczema or a perfectly healthy skin, it makes sense to make your own soap. Far from being a chore, it is actually a great deal of fun and it can help your skin to stay radiant and healthy for a lot longer.

I have included recipes in this book for you to try but I will also share how to make your very own recipes from scratch. I urge you to experiment and play around with soap crafting until you get the results that you are aiming for.

Choose your own custom ingredients and scents to use. I, for example, hate the smell of Tea Tree oil so I never use it in any of my soaps at all. One of my cousins, on the other hand, loves the smell. We are all different, with different likes and dislikes.

Making your own soap, to your own preferences, is a really fun and liberating experience.

And it is a lot friendlier to the environment as well because we are using only natural ingredients. We are not bothering with synthetic fragrance oils and colorants.

And, as if you needed any further encouragement, this is a cost-effective and practical way to express your individuality.

You may ask why you should make your own soaps – I ask why would you not want to? If you want the very best for yourself and your family, and want to reduce the number of synthetic chemicals in your life, this is a great place to start.

Chapter 2: The Squeaky Clean Truth About Soaps

A brief history of soap

The soap has a remarkable past. For an extremely, long time, individuals have realized that joining fats with debris from a fire would make a substance that could be utilized to clean things. There is a broadly recounted story that the word soap originated from the antiquated Romans notwithstanding, the reality of it is generally discussed. As per the story, Romans relinquished creatures on Mount Sapo, and afterward it down-poured, the entirety of the fat from the creatures and the cinders from the conciliatory flames, were washed down the mountain and into the Tiber River. This made the earth in the stream that made washing simpler. Those that markdown this story as a dream has the conviction that the word soap gets from the Latin word, "Sapo" and was obtained from the Celts who made a substance from creature fat and plant debris that they called saipo.

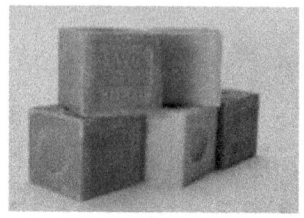

Antiquarians have a few thoughts regarding where and when soap making initially started. Many accept that soap was developed by the Babylonians. This is because a stone tablet was found during an uncovering of old Babylonia demonstrating that around 2800 B.C., Babylonians were making soap. Another sign that soap has been around since antiquated occasions are the Eber's papyrus which contains a formula for a soap made by salt blended in with creature fats showing that early Egyptians utilized soap for materials and restorative purposes. Early Romans made soap in the first century A.D. by consolidating goat fat with wood remains and salt. Truth be told, a salt processing plant was found among the remains of Pompeii, a city that was annihilated by a volcanic emission in 79 A.D.

In the second century A.D., Galen, the renowned Greek specialist, freely prescribed washing with soap to forestall illness. Preceding this, the soap was utilized essentially to treat sicknesses or for materials. This decree brought about more individuals utilizing soap for washing notwithstanding, for quite a while still; soap was utilized generally for non-washing purposes.

Moving into Europe, antiquated German's made soap from debris and creature fat. It was utilized fundamentally for styling hair. In 1200 A.D., Marseilles, France, and Savona, Italy were soap making centers. In the eighth century, there is proof that individuals in Italy and Spain were utilizing goat fat and beech tree debris to make soap.

Simultaneously, the French started utilizing olive oil in their soap. Soap came to Bristol, England in the twelfth century and could be found in London in the thirteenth century. Starting in the sixteenth century, better, more rich soaps that were vegetable-based, most utilizing olive oil, were all the more broadly accessible in Europe. In England, soap producers needed to pay the charge on the soap that they made until 1853. This was authorized to the point of outfitting soap pots with locks so soap creators would not have the option to deliver soap without being watched. At the point when the expense was reduced, the modest soap was made and turned out to be generally accessible all through England by 1880.

In 1791, a Frenchman by the name of Nicolas LeBlanc found an approach to make sodium carbonate or soft drink debris from regular salt which permitted soap producers to make soap modestly. Before this, the soap was costly and in exceptional popularity. In 1811, another Frenchman named Michel Eugene Chevreul distinguished the connection between glycerin and unsaturated fats. These two revelations denoted the start of advanced soap making.

In the late eighteenth century, modernly made soap opened up be that as it may, up until around the transform into the nineteenth century, Europeans kept on utilizing soap principally for purposes other than washing. This changed when German scientific expert Justus Von Liebig declared that the measure of soap utilized by a country was an extraordinary pointer of the nation's riches and level of affability.

At the point when the primary pilgrims came to America, they carried a huge flexibly of soap with them. This can be confirmed by review the records of boats that came over from England. In 1630, John Winthrop, before he turned into the principal legislative head of the Massachusetts Bay Colony, kept in touch with his significant other requesting that she bring soap when she ventured out over to America. In the wake of building up themselves in America and enduring their first cruel winter, the pilgrims found that they had an enormous flexibly of debris and creature fat because of their day by day schedules of chasing and preparing food. They went to the acknowledgment that they could make soap from those items. At the point when they started doing this, the soap was not, at this point a costly item that was popular. It could be made for essentially no cash and was commonly made yearly or semiannually. For the pioneers, making their own soap had the additional advantage of permitting them to be progressively more autonomous of England.

In 1916, the soap making measure changed fundamentally when German scientists found and started making manufactured soaps. Monetarily made soap as we probably are aware it today opened up during World War I. Around then, processing plants were utilizing the group pot bubbling technique for making soap. This cycle had some noteworthy downsides. In addition to the fact that it took four to eleven days to finish a bunch, the nature of the created soap was conflicting and subject to which oils were utilized in a specific group. Soon after 1930, the Proctor and Gamble Company built up the consistent soap making measure. This change brought about the creation of a steady nature of soap that was made in a shorter measure of time. This cycle is as yet utilized by business organizations today and permits a bunch of soaps to be finished in around six hours.

What is a soap?

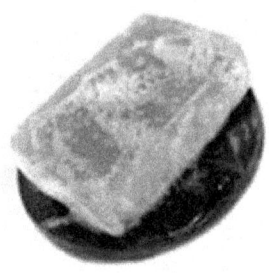

Before diving into the craft of soap making, we should initially see precisely what a soap is. A few people tend to skip parts, for example, this and make a plunge directly into the heading giving a segment of things. Be forewarned avoiding ahead to find out about what you have to accumulate to make your first group will be impeding. To make something it is basic that one comprehends the essentials to be effective. Since soap making is so experimentally based, when you comprehend the standards and speculations about how soap is shaped and why it framed, you will have the option to apply your learning not exclusively to following a formula however making your own novel and a shrewd show-stopper. You are out in front of the game on the off chance that you ever took a science class, so put on your sterile garment and read on.

In its most fundamental structure, the soap is essentially the salt of unsaturated fat. Actually no, not the sort of salt that we keep on our tables to sprinkle on French fries. A salt is whatever is the result of a corrosive and a soluble base responding. The kind of salt that is framed from this response is subject to the quality of the corrosive and antacid that is joining.

Review from science, the pH, or potential Hydrogen scale. On this scale, water is nonpartisan at a 7. Anything short of 7 is corrosive. Anything over 7 is a soluble base. At that point scale permits soluble bases and acids to be portrayed as solid or frail substances. More grounded acids tend to consume while more grounded salts tend to erode. The pH scale likewise gives us a perspective to test substances to guarantee that they are sheltered to be contacted or ingested.

With regards to soap, the corrosive that is utilized by and large comes as unsaturated fats got from creatures and plants. Every unsaturated fat has one hydrogen, two oxygen, and one-carbon iota and has a carboxylic corrosive gathering hanging out toward the end. This carboxylic corrosive gathering is comprised of hydrogen and carbon molecules. Presently, when unsaturated fats meet up, they connect themselves into gatherings of three and structure what is called fatty oil atoms. The fatty oil atom is likewise joined to one particle of glycerin. Cling to that data while we change gears a piece.

An antacid is a base that will kill a corrosive and break up in the water. At the point when salt and a corrosive blend, the balance of the two happens through the creation of hydrogen and oxygen particles during the response cycle. At the point when soap originally began being made, cinders of plants filled in as the salt that was utilized to cause a response with the unsaturated fats. In these advanced occasions, antacids are made financially. The soluble base that is utilized, only, in soap making is lye. Lye can be bought at a home improvement shop. It is otherwise called sodium hydroxide or acidic pop. Lye is alluded to as burning because of its inclination to be extremely destructive.

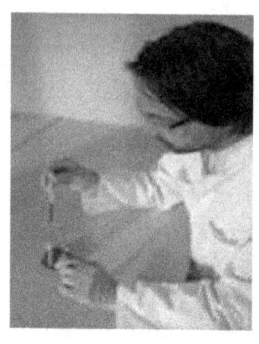

So now we realize that soap is a salt that is made when an unsaturated fat is joined with an antacid. We recognize what unsaturated fats and soluble bases are. Presently here comes the most significant soapmaking term you will actually learn. Submit it to memory. S-A-P-O-N-I-F-I-C-A-T-I-O-N. Saponification is the synthetic cycle of making soap. Here is the thing that occurs in essential terms. The salt attempts to part the unsaturated fats into two sections, unsaturated fats, and glycerin. At that point the salt ties with the unsaturated fat. So once saponification has happened, we are left with a tablet of salt and glycerin.

You may now be pondering, so if we are left with salt and glycerin, how precisely does that spotless thing? Well, that is more science. At the point when the soap is joined with water, it goes about as a surfactant. A surfactant particle has oil dissolvable and water solvent parts. Along these lines, these atoms can encompass oil or earth particles and carry them into the water so they can be washed away.

Alright. Since you have the entirety of that foundation data put away in your cerebrum you are prepared to find out about how soaps are made. There are commonly four cycles that can be utilized to make handcrafted soap. You can decide to utilize the virus cycle, the hot cycle, they soften and pour technique or the rebatching strategy. Every one of these strategies will be clarified in detail as you read on. They all share something practically speaking in any case, and that is the saponification cycle that needs to happen at some point, in one way or another to make soap. So you will consistently require an oil or fat and a basic (quite often lye) to make a traditional soap.

The soap making procedure

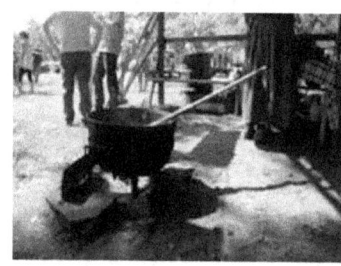

There are a few distinct techniques that can be utilized to make soaps nowadays. We will examine these strategies in a lot more prominent detail in later parts yet the cycle merits an outline now. The soap making ceremonial starts with mixing two separate creations. The first is a mix of lye and water. The second is a mix of fats and oils. These two arrangements are combined until a point called to follow is reached. Follow is where enough saponification has happened that the blend has begun to thicken. When all is said in done, when follow happens the soap is filled a shape or the like. Contingent upon the strategy for soap making being utilized, the soap will at that point experience a gel stage where it turns out to be mistier in shading. A gel stage doesn't generally happen and doesn't really need to happen. At the point when a portion of log shape is utilized, the gel stage will in general happen because the blend holds its warmth well and will condense while in the form. Soaps that are filled individual molds don't will in general hold their warmth too and along these lines are not as prone to experience the gel stage. On the off chance that a soap experiences a gel stage, saponification will in general be quicker. Regardless of whether it experiences a gel stage or not, after the soap has solidified in the form, it is taken out and put on racks to fix. The relieving cycle takes around 3 a month and a half to finish and permits the soap to solidify and age. In the wake of relieving is finished the soap is prepared to utilize.

You may review from prior that the pot clump measure is one way that organizations used to make exceptionally a lot of soap. This is a four-venture measure which is plot straightaway.

Boiling

In this initial step, the fats and the soluble base are dissolved into a huge steel pot. A huge organization may have a pot that is three stories tall and can hold a few thousand pounds of fixings. Warmth curls inside the pot heat the blend to bubbling. Saponification starts as the fats and antacid blend, creating soap and glycerin.

Salting

In request to isolate the glycerin and soap, salt is added to the blend. At the point when the salt is included, the soap ascends to the head of the pot and glycerin settles to the base. The glycerin is taken out through the base of the pot.

Strong change

A burning arrangement is then added to the pot during what is alluded to as the solid change stage to eliminate any fats that have not saponified. This is critical to accomplishing a soap that is smooth and liberated from debasements. The blend is bubbled again and the fat goes to soap. Salting can be rehashed now if essential.

Pitching

In this last advance, water is added to the pot and the soap is brought to one more bubble. The blend will isolate into two layers after time. The top layer, containing about 70% soap and 30% water, is alluded to as "perfect soap". The base later contains the rest of the water, earth, and different polluting influences. This layer is classified as "nigre". The soap is shaped, cooled, and restored before it is wrapped and prepared for procurement.

The most current technique used to mass-produce soap is the Continuous Process. It works this way:

Splitting

This initial step parts the fat being utilized to make the soap into unsaturated fats and glycerin. The cycle happens in a tall treated steel section called a hydrolyzed. Fat is siphoned into one finish of the section and high temp water is siphoned into the opposite end. The section is then profoundly pressurized. As the parting cycle happens, the unsaturated fats and the glycerin are siphoned out of the section while simultaneously more fat and water are added to the segment. The eliminated unsaturated fats are then purged through a refining cycle to guarantee that they are smooth and liberated from debasements.

Mixing

A soluble base is currently blended in with the cleaned unsaturated fats to deliver soap. Added substances, for example, shading, aroma, and exfoliators are placed into the blend during this progression.

Cooling and Finishing

The soap is filled forms and solidifies into a huge piece. Coolers are in some cases used to accelerate this cycle. Bars of soap is then cut from the chunk and wrapped.

Since you have a decent foundation of what soap is and its history just as an essential comprehension of how it is made, the time has come to dig in more profound and begin figuring out how to make your own soap.

Chapter 3: Simple Soap Recipes

Melt-And-Pour Soap Recipes

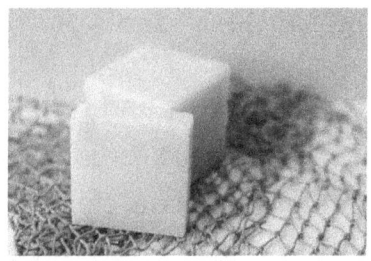

Apple Pie Soap

This soap smells delicious and makes for a great holiday gift.

Ingredients

1 lb. shea melt-and-pour soap base

0.25 oz. (½ tbsp.) vanilla extract

0.16 oz. (1 tsp.) Apple fragrance oil

½ tsp. cinnamon

red liquid colorant

Instructions

Cut the soap base into small cubes and place them in a microwave-safe bowl. Microwave in 30-second increments, stirring after each burst.

Once soap base has completely melted, add 1 to 2 drops of colorant and mix until you're satisfied with the color. Add the vanilla extract, cinnamon, and fragrance oil. Mix thoroughly.

Pour soap into the cavities of your mold. Spritz some alcohol on the surface if there are bubbles on your soap.

Allow the soap to cool and completely harden for at least 2 hours before removing from the mold.

Black Raspberry Soap

This melt-and-pour exfoliating soap is perfect for beginners. It only requires 4 ingredients and you could substitute the raspberry seeds with any exfoliant you already have, like poppy seeds. You could also swap out the madder root with any natural colorant, like paprika and turmeric.

Ingredients

1 lb. olive oil melt-and-pour soap base

0.16 oz. (1 tsp.) black raspberry scented oil

½ tsp. raspberry seeds

½ tsp. madder root powder

Instructions

Cut the soap base into small pieces using a kitchen knife. Place them in a microwave-safe container. Melt the soap in the microwave at 30-second intervals, stirring after each increment. Microwave until soap is fully melted.

Stir in the raspberry oil, raspberry seeds, and madder root. Mix until color is fully incorporated.

Pour soap mixture into the mold. Set aside for 2 hours or until soap is firm.

When the soap has completely hardened and cooled, remove it from the mold.

Cinnamon Soap

If you want to make an excellent handmade gift for men, try this recipe.

Ingredients

1 lb. clear melt-and-pour soap base

0.08 oz. (½ tsp.) cinnamon essential oil

1 tbsp. poppy seeds

red liquid colorant

Instructions

Cut the soap base into small cubes and place them in a microwave-safe bowl. Melt the soap in the microwave at 30-second intervals, stirring in between bursts.

Once the soap base has completely melted, stir in the essential oil. Add the poppy seeds and a drop or two of colorant. Mix until color is fully dispersed. Feel free to add more colorant until you're satisfied with the color.

Pour the soap mixture into your prepared mold. Lightly spray with alcohol to get rid of bubbles.

Set the soap aside for at least 2 hours to cool and harden. Remove soap from the mold after it has fully hardened.

Cranberry Vanilla Soap

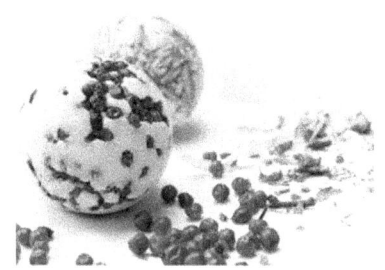

This soap has a soft vanilla scent. The dried cranberries give it some holiday feel.

Ingredients

1 lb. shea melt-and-pour soap base

¼ cup dried cranberries

0.04 oz. (20 drops) vanilla soap fragrance

Instructions

Divide the dried cranberries evenly between the cavities of your mold. Set aside.

Cut the soap base into small cubes and place them in a microwave-safe bowl. Melt them in the microwave in 30-second increments, stirring in between each burst.

Once the soap base has completely melted, stir in the essential oil. Mix thoroughly.

Pour the melted soap into your prepared mold. Lightly spray the soap with alcohol to get rid of bubbles.

Set the soap aside for at least 2 hours to cool and harden before removing from the mold.

Earl Grey Tea Soap

Infused with citrus essential oils, this melt-and-pour soap smells wonderful. This recipe uses a triple butter soap base, giving the soap a lovely lather.

Ingredients

2 lbs. triple butter melt-and-pour soap base

0.16 oz. (1 tsp.) bergamot essential oil

0.08 oz. (½ tsp.) Litsea cubeba essential oil

0.08 oz. (½ tsp.) sweet orange essential oil

2 tea bags of earl grey tea

Instructions

Cut the soap base into small chunks and place them in a microwave-safe bowl. Melt the soap in the microwave using 30-second intervals, stirring in between.

Once the soap base has completely melted, add 1 bag of tea and mix thoroughly. Stir in the essential oils and mix until they're fully dispersed.

Pour the soap mixture into your prepared mold. Spritz some alcohol on the surface if there are bubbles on your soap. Sprinkle the other bag of tea evenly on top of the soap.

Set the soap aside for 2 to 4 hours to cool and harden. When the soap has fully hardened, remove it from the mold and slice into bars, if necessary.

Flower Cupcake Soap

These flower cupcake soaps are made easy using melt-and-pour soap base. You won't need to add color to make them look stunning but you can definitely use some light colorant if you want to. For this recipe, you'll have to use small paper or silicone cupcake cases to shape the soap.

Ingredients

1 lb. white melt-and-pour soap base

0.4 oz. (2.5 tsp.) fragrance oil

dried rose petals

Instructions

Chop the soap base into small pieces and place them in a microwave-safe dish. Microwave the soap base in 30-second increments, stirring after each interval.

Once the soap base has fully melted, add the fragrance oil and mix thoroughly. Pour soap into the cupcake cases, leaving about ½" of a gap at the top. Make sure that you leave enough soap for the top layer.

Set the soap aside to harden slightly so the petals won't sink when they're added. Once the tops are firm enough to hold a thin layer of soap, lightly spray each with alcohol. Add some soap to each cupcake case and sprinkle with the dried petals.

Allow the soaps to completely dry for a few hours before removing them from the case.

Gingerbread Soap

This easy-to-make soap is a great homemade holiday gift. For this recipe, you need a 6-cavity gingerbread man mold.

Ingredients

16 oz. white melt-and-pour soap base

0.25 oz. (½ tbsp.) gingerbread fragrance oil

brown sparkle color bar

Instructions

Chop the soap base into small chunks. Melt the soap in the microwave using 30-second bursts, stirring in between.

Once melted, add a small amount of the color bar and mix thoroughly. Add more in small amounts until you're satisfied with the color.

Add the fragrance oil and stir until fully dispersed.

Pour the soap mixture into your prepared mold. Spray soap with alcohol if there are bubbles. Set aside to cool and harden. Remove from the mold after the soap has fully hardened.

Goat's Milk Lemon Soap

Here's a simple recipe that you and your kids will enjoy making.

Ingredients

2 lbs. goat's milk melt-and-pour soap base

0.5 oz. (3 tsp.) lemon essential oil

lemon (or another citrus, like lime and orange)

Instructions

Choose lemon that's small enough to fit the size of your mold. Slice it into 1/8" rounds. Place a wire rack on a pan and lay the slices on top of it. Leave it inside your oven preheated to 200°F for 2 to 3 hours or until the lemon is dry. Remove the dried slices and set them aside to cool.

Cut the goat's milk soap base into small pieces and place them in a microwave-safe container. Microwave at 30-second intervals, stirring in between. Once the soap is completely melted, add the essential oil and stir.

While the soap base is in the microwave, lay out the dried lemon slices inside the cavities of your mold.

Quickly pour the melted soap into the mold. After a few hours, pop the soap out of the mold.

Grapefruit Soap With Himalayan Salt

Here's a quick and easy way to incorporate Himalayan salt into your soap. This recipe is so simple it only requires 3 ingredients.

Ingredients

1 lb. goat's milk melt-and-pour soap base

0.04 oz. (¼ tsp.) grapefruit essential oil

¼ cup pink Himalayan salt

Instructions

Cut the soap base into small chunks and place them in a microwave-safe bowl. Melt the soap in 30-second intervals, stirring in between.

Once the soap base has completely melted, stir in the essential oil. Add the Himalayan salt and mix until they're evenly dispersed.

Pour the soap mixture into the cavities of your prepared mold. Lightly spray with alcohol to get rid of bubbles.

Set the soap aside for at least 2 hours to cool and harden before removing them from the mold.

Honey And Oatmeal Soap

This simple recipe is perfect for all beginners. It's quite easy to make and the ingredients are easily accessible if you don't have them yet in your kitchen.

Ingredients

1 lb. Castile or glycerin melt-and-pour soap base

½ oz. 100% pure honey

4 tbsp. steel-cut oatmeal

Instructions

Cut the soap base into small cubes and place them in a stockpot or a large saucepan. Using a stove burner, melt the soap over medium heat. Stir once in a while until soap is fully melted but don't allow it to boil. Remove pan from heat.

Place the honey in a small microwave-safe bowl. Put it in the microwave on high for 15 seconds. Immediately pour the heated honey into the melted soap base and stir until the two ingredients are combined well.

Add oatmeal to the mixture. Stir until oats are evenly distributed.

Pour the soap mixture into the cavities of your prepared mold. Spritz some alcohol on the surface if there are bubbles forming on your soap.

Set the soap aside for 2 to 4 hours to cool and harden before removing them from the mold.

Honeysuckle Soap

This soap recipe will allow you to enjoy the scent of honeysuckle year round. The turmeric powder gives this soap a natural color.

Ingredients

2 lbs. baby buttermilk melt-and-pour soap base

0.75 oz. (4.5 tsp.) wild honeysuckle fragrance oil

½ tsp. turmeric powder

0.1 oz. vitamin E oil (optional)

Instructions

Chop the soap base into small chunks. Melt them in the microwave. Don't forget to stir every 30 seconds.

Once melted, add the turmeric powder and mix until fully incorporated. Make sure no clumps of powder remain.

Stir in the fragrance oil and vitamin E oil. Mix thoroughly.

Pour the soap into your prepared mold. If there are any bubbles, lightly spray the soap with isopropyl alcohol.

Set the soap aside to cool and harden. After about 2 hours, remove soap from the mold.

Lemon Poppy Seed Soap

The soap base for this recipe is infused with 3 kinds of butter—mango, shea, and cocoa. But this recipe will work with any kind of soap base.

Ingredients

1 lb. triple butter melt-and-pour soap base

0.16 oz. (1 tsp.) lemon fragrance oil

2 tbsp. poppy seeds

½ tsp. yellow soap colorant

Instructions

Using a kitchen knife, cut the soap base into small cubes and place them in a microwave-safe bowl. Melt the cubes in the microwave using 30-second intervals. Stir soap between each interval.

Once soap base has completely melted, add the colorant a few drops at a time and stir thoroughly until the color is completely incorporated and you've achieved the tone you want.

Stir in the fragrance oil and mix to disperse. Add the poppy seeds and stir thoroughly. You can use less or more seeds depending on how you want your soap to look.

Pour soap into the loaf mold. Continue stirring until it thickens to keep the seeds from settling at the bottom. Set aside for a couple of hours to cool and harden.

Remove soap from the mold and slice it into bars.

Lime And Cilantro Soap

The combination of lime and cilantro essential oils gives this soap an invigorating scent.

Ingredients

1 lb. shea melt-and-pour soap base

0.04 oz. (¼ tsp.) lime essential oil

0.04 oz. (¼ tsp.) cilantro essential oil

Instructions

Cut the soap base into small chunks and place them in a microwave-safe bowl. Microwave in 30-second intervals, stirring after each burst until soap melts completely.

Add the essential oils to melted soap. Mix thoroughly.

Pour soap in the cavities of your prepared mold. If there are bubbles, spray the soap with isopropyl alcohol.

Allow soap to cool and harden for about 2 hours before removing from the mold.

Lemon And Raspberry Soap

Here's another simple recipe that you should try if you love the smell of citrus and raspberry. The added shea butter makes this soap extra-moisturizing.

Ingredients

1 lb. goat's milk melt-and-pour soap base

0.5 oz. (1 tbsp.) shea butter

0.08 (½ tsp.) lemon essential oil

0.08 (½ tsp.) raspberry essential oil

Instructions

Cut the soap base into small cubes. Melt the soap in the microwave, stirring after every 30 seconds.

Melt the shea butter in a separate container using 10-seconds bursts. Once melted, add it to the soap base.

Stir in the essential oils. Mix until they're fully dispersed.

Pour the soap mixture into your prepared mold. Spray soap with alcohol if there are bubbles. Set aside to cool and harden.

After about 2 hours or when the soap has fully hardened, remove it from the mold.

Lemongrass Soap

This recipe combines the healing properties of eucalyptus and the uplifting scent of lemongrass. Matcha powder gives the soap a natural green color.

Ingredients

1 lb. glycerin melt-and-pour soap base

0.5 oz. (1 tbsp.) shea butter

0.16 oz. (1 tsp.) lemongrass essential oil

0.08 oz. (½ tsp.) eucalyptus essential oil

0.08 oz. (½ tsp.) cedarwood essential oil

1 tsp. matcha powder

Instructions

Cut the soap base into small chunks and place them in a microwave-safe bowl. Melt the soap in 30-second intervals, stirring in between. Once melted, add the shea butter and heat until it melts.

Add matcha powder to the melted soap and mix until it completely dissolves into the soap. Stir in the essential oil and mix to disperse.

Pour the soap mixture into your prepared mold. Lightly spray with alcohol if there are bubbles.

Set the soap aside for at least 2 hours. Remove soap from the mold after it has completely hardened.

Milk And Honey Soap

This quick-and-easy recipe creates a soap that offers lots of skin benefits. To make your soap look unique, use a silicone honeycomb mold.

Ingredients

1 lb. goat's milk melt-and-pour soap base

2.25 oz. raw honey

liquid soap colorant (optional)

Instructions

Slice the soap base into small cubes using a kitchen knife. Place the cubes in a microwave-safe container. Cover the container to keep the soap from drying out.

Melt the soap in the microwave with 30-second intervals, stirring after each increment. Make sure soap is completely melted before proceeding to the next step.

Stir in raw honey and a few drops of the colorant of your choice.

Pour soap mixture into the mold and set aside for at least two hours.

When the soap has completely hardened and cooled, remove it from the mold.

Orange And Bergamot Soap

This recipe uses essential oils that give the soap a soothing and sweet smell. Paprika gives it a natural orange color.

Ingredients

1 lb. white melt-and-pour soap base

1 tsp. paprika powder

0.16 oz. (1 tsp.) bergamot essential oil

0.16 oz. (1 tsp.) sweet orange essential oil

0.04 oz. (¼ tsp.) frankincense essential oil

Instructions

Cut the soap base into small cubes and place them in a microwave-safe bowl. Melt the soap in 30-second intervals, stirring in between each burst.

Once the soap base has completely melted, add the paprika powder. Mix until fully dissolved and the color is evenly dispersed. Stir in the essential oils and mix thoroughly.

Pour the soap mixture into your prepared mold. Lightly spray with isopropyl alcohol to get rid of bubbles.

Set the soap aside for at least 2 hours to cool and harden before removing from the mold.

Orange Turmeric Soap

This beginner-friendly recipe uses turmeric to give color to the soap. The orange scent perfectly complements the natural orange color.

Ingredients

2 lbs. goat's milk melt-and-pour soap base

1 tsp. turmeric powder

0.4 oz. (2.5 tsp.) orange essential oil

1 tbsp. 99% isopropyl alcohol

Instructions

Combine the turmeric powder and isopropyl alcohol and mix. This helps the turmeric powder disperse into the soap without lumps. Set aside.

Cut the soap base into small cubes and place them in a microwave-safe bowl. Melt the soap in the microwave using 30-second intervals, stirring between each burst.

Once the soap base has completely melted, stir in the essential oil and dispersed turmeric. Mix thoroughly.

Pour the soap mixture into a 6-cavity rectangular mold. Lightly spray the top of each bar with isopropyl alcohol if there are bubbles.

Set the soap aside for at least 2 hours to cool and harden. When the soap has fully hardened, remove the bars from the mold.

Patchouli Charcoal Soap

If you want a detoxifying facial soap, you can easily make one with this recipe.

Ingredients

1.5 oz. shea butter melt-and-pour soap base

2 tbsp. activated charcoal powder

0.16 oz. (1 tsp.) patchouli essential oil

Instructions

Cut the soap base into small cubes and melt them in the microwave in 30-second intervals. Stir soap in between each burst.

Once the soap base has completely melted, add the activated charcoal powder. Mix until the color is evenly dispersed and no clumps of charcoal remain. Stir in the essential oil and mix thoroughly.

Pour the soap mixture into your prepared mold. If there are any bubbles, lightly spray the soap with isopropyl alcohol.

Set the soap aside for at least 2 hours to cool and harden before removing from the mold.

Pumpkin Spice Soap

This recipe is for a lightly colored soap. If you want your soap to have a brighter color, feel free to add a few more drops of colorant.

Ingredients

2 lbs. shea butter melt-and-pour soap base

2 tbsp. pumpkin pie spice

4 drops yellow colorant

2 drops red colorant

Instructions

Cut the soap base into small chunks and place them in a microwave-safe bowl. Melt the soap in 30-second intervals, stirring in between.

Once the soap base has completely melted, stir in the pumpkin pie spice and colorant. Mix until they're fully dispersed.

Pour the soap mixture into your prepared mold. If there are bubbles forming on your soap, lightly spray it with alcohol.

Set the soap aside for at least 2 hours to cool and harden. When the soap has fully hardened, remove it from the mold and slice into bars.

Rose Loofah Soap

Loofah soaps naturally exfoliate, allowing moisture to fully nourish the skin. They make great handmade gifts for many occasions. For this project, you need to find a mold that's big enough to fit the loofah.

Ingredients

1 lb. goat's milk or avocado melt-and-pour soap base

0.03 oz. (15 drops) rose essential oil

½ tsp. rose mica powder

1 natural loofah

Instructions

Cut loofah into 1" rounds. If you want the loofah completely inside your soap, make thinner slices. Place the slices in the mold.

Mix mica powder with a small amount of alcohol. Set aside.

Break the soap base into small chunks and place them in a microwave-safe bowl. Microwave on 30-second intervals until soap is completely melted, stirring in between intervals.

Add the mica to the melted soap. Continue to mix until color is evenly dispersed. Stir in the essential oil.

Pour soap in the mold. If there are bubbles forming, spray it lightly with isopropyl alcohol. Set aside.

Remove the soap from the mold after a couple of hours.

Spiced Apple Soap

This simple soap recipe uses apple spice and fragrance oil for a lovely scent of fall.

Ingredients

1 lb. goat's milk melt-and-pour soap base

0.16 oz. (1 tsp.) Apple fragrance oil

½ tsp. apple pie spice

orange liquid soap colorant

Instructions

Cut the soap base into small chunks and place them in a microwave-safe bowl. Melt soap in the microwave using 30-second intervals, stirring after each burst.

Once melted, stir in the apple pie spice and essential oil. Add 2 drops of orange colorant and mix thoroughly.

Pour soap into your prepared mold. If you see any bubbles, spray the soap with isopropyl alcohol to get rid of them.

Set aside for about 2 hours. Release the soap bars from the mold after they have completely hardened.

Sweet Almond Soap

This simple recipe makes a mildly-scented soap that softens and lightly exfoliates the skin.

Ingredients

1 lb. shea butter melt-and-pour soap base

0.16 oz. (1 tsp.) sweet almond fragrance oil

1 tbsp. poppy seeds

Instructions

Cut the soap base into small chunks and place them in a microwave-safe bowl. Melt the soap in 30-second intervals, stirring in between.

Once the soap base has completely melted, stir in the essential oil and poppy seeds. Mix until they're fully dispersed.

Pour the soap mixture into your prepared mold. If there are bubbles, lightly spray the soap with alcohol.

Set the soap aside for at least 2 hours to cool and harden. Pop the soap out of the mold after it has fully hardened.

Vanilla Latte Soap

Love coffee? This soap recipe is for you.

Ingredients

1 lb. goat's milk melt-and-pour soap base

coffee grounds (for 1 cup of coffee)

vanilla essential oil

Instructions

Brew a cup of coffee. Set aside both coffee and grounds.

Cut the soap base into small chunks and place them in a microwave-safe bowl. Place the bowl in the microwave and melt the soap in 30-second intervals, stirring in between.

Once the soap base has completely melted, add the coffee grounds, a ¼ cup of the brewed coffee, and a few drops of essential oil. Mix until they're fully dispersed.

Pour the soap mixture into your prepared mold. If there are bubbles forming on your soap, lightly spray it with alcohol.

Set the soap aside for at least 2 hours to cool and harden. When the soap bars have fully hardened, remove them from the mold.

White Tea And Ginger Loofah Soap

Here's another loofah soap recipe, but this time it has a white tea and ginger scent. You may also want to use a round silicone soap mold that's about the size of your loofah.

Ingredients

1 lb. detergent-free glycerin melt-and-pour soap base

0.4 oz. (3 tsp.) white tea and ginger fragrance oil

liquid soap colorant (optional)

1 loofah

Instructions

Using a bread knife, slice the loofah into 1" rounds. Place the loofah rounds into each cavity of the mold.

Cut the soap base into small cubes using a kitchen knife. Place the cubes in a Pyrex measuring cup and microwave in 30-second increments until soap has fully melted, stirring in between.

Stir fragrance oil into the soap base. Add the liquid colorant a few drops at a time and mix until color is fully incorporated and you're satisfied with the hue.

Pour the soap into the cavities of your mold. The loofah will absorb some of the melted soap so you'll have to pour more soap until each cavity is filled completely.

Set the soap aside for a few hours to harden. When it's hard enough, pop each soap out of the mold.

Cold-Process Soap Recipes

Castile Soap

Castile soaps are made purely with . It's so easy to make but the soap will take a lot more time to completely harden.

Ingredients

16 oz. olive oil

4.8 oz. distilled water

2.06 oz. lye

½ oz. sodium lactate (optional)

Instructions

Place the water in a heat-proof container. Slowly add the lye and stir until it has totally dissolved. Set aside and allow the solution to cool to around 110°F. Stir in sodium lactate when the temperature reaches below 130°F.

Heat the olive oil up to around 110°F in the microwave or in a pot over low heat.

Once the right temperature is reached, carefully pour the lye solution to the olive oil. Blend using a stick blender. Alternate between manually stirring and pulsing, then bring the mixture to a medium trace. This will take several minutes.

Pour the soap batter into your prepared mold. Cover the mold with a piece of cardboard and towel to insulate the soap.

After 24 to 48 hours, check if the soap has completely hardened. If not, give it more time in the mold but without the cover. Once the soap is firm enough, remove it from the mold. Cut into bars, if necessary. Allow soap to cure for 4 to 6 weeks.

Coconut Soap

Requiring only three ingredients, this is definitely among the simplest soap recipes. It's the perfect recipe if you want to try making cold-process soap.

Ingredients

33 oz. coconut oil

9.6 oz. water

4.83 oz. lye

0.8 oz. fragrance oil (optional)

Instructions

Place cold water in a heat-proof container. Slowly add the lye and stir until it has totally dissolved. Set aside and allow the solution to cool.

Melt coconut oil in a large pan over low heat. Once it has melted, remove from heat and allow to cool.

Once the temperatures are at 100-110°F, carefully pour the lye solution to the melted coconut oil. Blend using a stick blender, alternating between manually mixing and pulsing. If you're adding fragrance oil, bring the mixture to a light trace. Otherwise, blend to a medium trace.

Add the fragrance or essential oil of your choice to the soap mixture. Blend until completely mixed and bring the mixture to a medium trace.

Pour soap mixture into your prepared mold. Cover the mold with a piece of cardboard and insulate the soap by covering it with a towel.

If your soap needs to be cut into bars, remove it from the mold once it has cooled and hardened. Don't wait for 24 hours or it will be too hard to cut. Allow the bars to cure for 2 to 3 weeks.

Lard Soap

If it's your first time making a cold-process soap, this is the perfect recipe. It uses 100% lard, which is cheap and easy to find.

Ingredients

2 lbs. lard

12.16 oz. distilled water

4.25 oz. lye

0.8 oz. fragrance oil (optional)

Instructions

Place the water in a heatproof container. Slowly add the lye and stir until it has totally dissolved. Set aside and allow the solution to cool to 110-120°F.

Melt the lard in a large pan over low heat. Once melted, remove from heat and allow to cool to 110-120°F.

Once the right temperature is reached, carefully pour the lye solution to the melted lard. Blend using a stick blender. Alternate between manually stirring and pulsing and bring the mixture to a light trace.

Stir in the fragrance oil, if using. Continue blending until the batter reaches a medium trace.

Pour the soap batter into the prepared mold. Insulate the soap for 24 hours by covering the mold with a piece of cardboard and towel.

Once the soap is firm enough, remove it from the mold. Cut soap into bars and let them cure for 4 to 6 weeks.

Basic Tallow Soap

Tallow is fat derived from cattle. Like lard, it's inexpensive and easy to find.

Ingredients

8 oz. tallow

4 oz. coconut oil

4 oz. olive oil

6.08 oz. water

2.27 oz. lye

Instructions

Place water in a heat-proof container. Slowly add the lye and stir until it completely dissolves. Set aside and allow the solution to cool to 110-120°F.

Melt tallow and coconut oil in a large pan over low heat. Once melted, add the olive oil. Remove from heat and allow to cool to 110-120°F.

Once the two mixtures reach the right temperature, carefully pour the lye solution into the oil mix. Blend using a stick blender. Alternate between manually stirring and pulsing, then bring the mixture to a medium trace.

Pour the soap batter into your prepared mold. Insulate the soap for 24 hours by covering the mold with a piece of cardboard and towel.

Remove soap from the mold and slice into bars. Allow bars to cure for 4 to 6 weeks.

Tallow Soap With Honey

This is a variation of the basic tallow soap recipe. The added honey imparts a light, sweet scent and helps increase the lather.

Ingredients

20 oz. tallow

4 oz. coconut oil

1 oz. honey

9.12 oz. distilled water

3.41 oz. lye

Instructions

Place water in a heatproof container. Slowly add the lye and stir until it has totally dissolved. Set aside and allow the solution to cool (100-110°F).

Place tallow and coconut oil in a pot over low heat. Once both are completely melted, add the honey. Remove from heat and allow to cool to 100-110°F.

Once the two mixtures reach the right temperature, carefully pour the lye solution into the oil mix. Blend using a stick blender. Alternate between manual stirring and pulsing until the mixture reaches a medium trace.

Pour soap mixture into your prepared mold and allow it to cool and harden. After 24 hours, remove soap from the mold and slice it into bars. Cure the soap bars for at least 4 weeks.

Basic Cold-Process Soap

Here's another cold process soap recipe that's great for beginners. It only requires 5 ingredients and the oils make the soap harden relatively fast.

Ingredients

26 oz. olive oil

6 oz. coconut oil

1 oz. castor oil

10 oz. water

4.4 oz. lye

Instructions

Place the water in a glass or sturdy plastic jug. Slowly add the lye and stir until it has totally dissolved. Set aside and allow the solution to cool.

Place the olive oil, coconut oil, and castor oil in a large pan and melt them over low heat. Remove from heat and allow to cool.

Once the temperatures of the two mixtures are at 90-100°F, carefully pour the lye solution to the oil mix. Blend using a stick blender and bring the mixture to a medium trace.

Pour soap mixture into the mold. If bubbles have formed, lightly spray the top with isopropyl alcohol to remove them.

Insulate the soap for 24 hours by covering the mold with a piece of cardboard and towel. Once it's firm enough, remove soap from the mold and let them cure for 3 to 4 weeks.

Basic Vegan Soap

Many handmade soap recipes include animal-based ingredients but it's not difficult to make a plant-based soap that's just as good. Here's a simple recipe for a cruelty-free soap.

Ingredients

16 oz. palm oil

16 oz. coconut oil

13.5 oz. olive oil

16 oz. water

6.5oz. lye

1 oz. fragrance or essential oil (optional)

Instructions

Place cooled water in a glass or sturdy plastic jug. Slowly add the lye and stir until it has totally dissolved. Set aside and allow the solution to cool.

Place the olive oil, coconut oil, and palm oil in a large pan and melt them over low heat. Once solid oils have melted, remove from heat and allow to cool.

Once the temperatures of the two mixtures are at 90-100°F, carefully pour the lye solution into the oil mix. Blend using a stick blender and bring the mixture to a light trace.

Add the fragrance or essential oil of your choice to the soap mixture. Blend until completely mixed and bring the mixture to a medium trace.

Pour soap mixture into the mold. Insulate the soap for 24 to 48 hours by covering the mold with a piece of cardboard and towel. Once it's firm enough, remove soap from the mold and let them cure for 3 to 4 weeks.

Bastille Soap

This recipe creates a soap with the same mildness as castile soap. It makes use of other oils to save some time. Colorful dried flowers are added, making them look more attractive.

Ingredients

20 oz. olive oil

2.5 oz. palm oil

2.5 oz. coconut oil

8 oz. water

3.25 oz. lye

0.5 oz. lavender fragrance oil (optional)

dried lavender flowers (optional)

Instructions

Slowly add the lye to the water and stir until the lye has totally dissolved. Set aside and allow the solution to cool to 100-110°F.

Place the olive oil, coconut oil, and palm oil in a large pan over low heat. Remove from heat when solid oils have melted and allow to cool.

Once the temperatures of the two mixture are within 10° of each other, carefully pour the lye solution into the oil mix. Blend using a stick blender and bring the mixture to a light trace.

Stir in the fragrance oil with the stick blender and blend until completely mixed. Bring the mixture to a medium trace.

Pour soap mixture into the mold. Remove any bubbles and prevent soda ash from forming by lightly spraying the top with 99% isopropyl alcohol.

Insulate the soap for 24 hours by covering the mold with a sheet of wax paper and a towel. Once it's firm enough, remove soap from the mold. If you're using a loaf mold, cut your soap into bars. Firmly press the top of each soap into the dried flowers and shake off any loose petals. Cure the soap bars for at least 4 weeks.

Supermarket Soap

This cold-process soap requires 4 oils, which you can easily find in any supermarket.

Ingredients

7.5 oz. olive oil

6.5 oz. palm oil

6.5 oz. coconut oil

1.3 oz. castor oil

8 oz. water

3.1 oz. lye

0.5 oz. fragrance or essential oil (optional)

Instructions

Place the water in a heatproof container. Slowly add the lye and stir until it has completely dissolved. Set aside and allow the solution to cool.

Place the coconut oil and palm oil in a pot over low heat. Once melted, add the olive oil and castor oil. Remove from heat and allow the mixture to cool.

Once the temperatures of the two mixtures reach 100-110°F, carefully pour the lye solution into the oil mix. Blend using a stick blender. Alternate between pulsing and manually stirring until the mixture reaches a light trace.

Stir in the fragrance oil and bring the mixture to a medium trace.

Pour the soap batter into your prepared mold. Insulate soap by covering the mold with a piece of cardboard and a towel. After 24 hours or when it has fully hardened, release it from the mold. Cut the soap into bars and let them cure for around 4 weeks.

Supermarket Soap With Shea Butter

This recipe uses 3 easy-to-find oils. The addition of shea butter makes the soap extra hydrating.

Ingredients

4.8 oz. olive oil

4.8 oz. coconut oil

3.2 oz. palm oil

3.2 oz. shea butter

6 oz. water

2.2 oz. lye

0.4 oz. fragrance or essential oil (optional)

Instructions

Place water in a heatproof container. Slowly add the lye and stir until it completely dissolves. Set aside and allow the solution to cool.

Place the coconut oil, palm oil, and shea butter in a pot over low heat. Once melted, add the olive oil. Remove from heat and allow the mixture to cool.

Once the temperatures of the two mixtures reach 100-110°F, carefully pour the lye solution into the oil mix. Blend using a stick blender. Alternate between pulsing and manually stirring until the mixture reaches a light trace.

Stir in the fragrance oil and bring the mixture to a medium trace.

Pour the soap batter into the cavities of your mold. Cover the mold with a piece of cardboard and a towel to insulate soap. After at least 24 hours, release the soap from the mold and cure for 4 to 6 weeks.

Lavender Soap

This simple soap recipe uses lavender essential oil for a soothing and relaxing scent.

Ingredients

14 oz. olive oil pomace

7 oz. coconut oil

7 oz. palm oil

10.64 oz. distilled water

3.94 lye

0.75 oz. lavender essential oil

Instructions

Place the water in a heatproof container. Slowly add the lye and stir until it has completely dissolved. Set aside and allow the solution to cool.

Place the coconut oil and palm oil in a pot over low heat. Once melted, add the olive oil. Remove from heat and allow the mixture to cool.

Once the temperatures of the two mixtures reach 100-110°F, carefully pour the lye solution into the oil mix. Blend using a stick blender. Alternate between pulsing and manually stirring until the mixture reaches a light trace.

Stir in the essential oil and bring the mixture to a medium trace.

Pour the soap batter into your prepared mold. Insulate soap by covering the mold with a piece of cardboard and a towel for 24 to 48 hours. Remove from the mold then cut into bars, if necessary. Allow the soap to cure for around 4 weeks.

Chapter 4: Equipment And Supplies Required

Whenever you are trying to make something be it cake, leather or my personal favorite, pancakes you need equipment to make your paste. For pancakes, for instance, you will require, a bowl, non-stick frying pan, cooking oil, flour and a mixer.

The same is applied to making soap. You need to have some equipment ready for you to make the soap, as well as safety supplies.

All the required supplies I will list them for you, to help you know what is necessary. They are quite cheap and you'd be surprised to note that you have some of them already in your house.

A heat resistant 3 to 5-quart container. The container has to be either plastic or stainless steel or an enamel covered pot and can be sealed. It will be used to mix your lye solution. An 8 to 12-quart container can be used if you want to make a large batch of soap.

A huge mixing pot that is either stainless steel or it can be an enamel covered pot. It is used to mix lye and it can be used to also melt base carrier oils as well. The container is to be used to mix all your ingredients together to get your batch of soap.

A food scale whose measurement units are both grams and ounces. You will use this to measure oils, lye, and water.

This equipment is crucial when making soap. To create a great bar of soap, the measurements must be perfect and precise. Weight over volume to have the reigns on what your soap should be.

Over time, the scale can start to show some irregularities, so to make it last longer and be able to survive after using essential oils on it for a long time here is a trick you can use: slide your scale into a larger gallon of plastic bag and seal the ends by using a packing tape. Oils won't affect the scale if they spill since it is protected.

Tightening the wrap or plastic bag on your scale is to make sure that wrinkles do not prevent you from seeing the digits displayed.

You can use a wrap instead of a plastic bag.

For stirring your lye mixture, have wooden or silicone spoons. Though you will be required to replace the wooden spoons, better have silicone utensils instead.

Rubber gloves and goggles are your safety equipment. This equipment is necessary when you are mixing lye or using it. Protect you skin and eyes ALWAYS when using lye. This is a precautionary measure that has to be taken, a MUST have. It is the same when you are dealing with caustic soap.

To heat your ingredients into liquid form, you are required to have a stainless-steel sauce pan. For instance, an ingredient that at room temperature is solid i.e. coconut oil, it requires heating before you use it.

Soap molds are a necessary equipment to make the shape of your soap, all dependent on what shape you want them to be like in the end. You can have PVC pipes or wooden loaf molds, and if you want fancy looking soaps have decorative molds.

When making several molds, you will need to have a soap cutter. Unless you want to use individual molds.

Soap making thermometers. Two of these to use for oil ingredients and the other for lye solution.

In case you have wooden mold, to avoid the soap from sticking to it you are going to need wax paper to line the mold with first.

Measuring spoons that will be used for your essential oils and colors. You can have custard cups to hold these ingredients to allow you to measure them properly.

To mix your colors, fragrance, and essential oils properly, get a small whisk.

Stick blender (there is a chance that you have got no clue what this is, I didn't either), but most recipes require you to have one. It is for blending oils and lye solution to allow saponification to begin, here is a picture of what the equipment looks like.

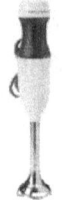

When you head out to get molds for your soap, choose molds that vary to have different shapes and make this process for you as much fun as possible. It is like shoe shopping, for your feet, but different types are the best...different molds for the same purpose.

Chapter 5: Natural Soap Making

Five Ways it Can Improve Your Life

I've noticed recently, most of my friends know nothing about natural soap making. When I tell people that I make my own soap - some are completely mystified, as if soap couldn't possibly be made anywhere but in an industrial lab, with expensive commercial equipment.

Nope! Not only can you make soap at home, but there are some fantastic benefits to doing so.

Here are my five favorite ways that learning to make your own soap can improve your life...

Give Yourself Gorgeous, Healthy Skin

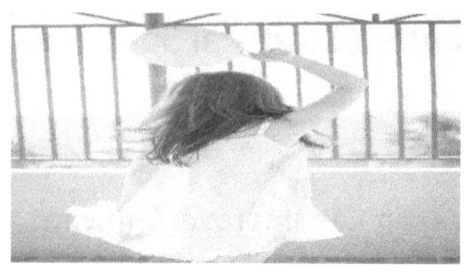

This is my favorite, because I never expected there to be SUCH a huge difference in how my skin felt, when I first tried homemade soap. Since I started using my own soap, I've gotten more compliments on my skin than you'd believe. The chronically dry skin that I once accepted as a bad draw from the gene pool has disappeared. My skin now *feels* good. It feels soft, smooth, and healthy. And healthy skin looks radiant and beautiful. Homemade soap is the easiest way in the world to give yourself great skin. I can't believe more people don't know about this. Natural soap that you make yourself has all the good stuff - the glycerin, oils, and moisturizers - that big companies strip out to resell. Make it yourself, and all you have to do is wash like normal - no change to your routine, no hours set aside for special beauty treatments - just shower, and voila, amazing skin that will have people asking, "what's your secret?"

Give Great Gifts

In the past, I struggled every year when the holidays came. I had so many people that felt close enough to give gifts too, but not so close that I instinctively knew what they'd love. And I hated the idea of giving yet another generic package of commercial soaps and lotions from the mall. Once I started making soap, this problem solved itself. Homemade soap wows your friends, because most people can't imagine being able to make it themselves. And, if they're wowed when they get it, just wait to see their reaction when they start using it! (A word of warning, don't be surprised if they start asking for more!)

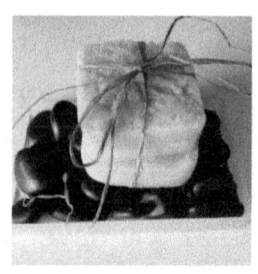

Start a Soap Business

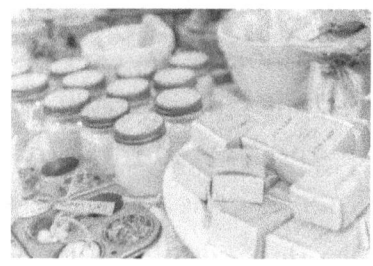

Looking for a little extra income in a tough economy? Or a way out of a bad job? Selling your own soaps can be done online, or locally at a farmer's market or flea market to help bring in some extra cash. How much you make will largely depend on the quality of your product, and how well you're able to bring in new customers. So brush up on your marketing skills, and get ready to roll!

Meet New Friends by Starting a Soap Club

Looking to meet new people, or connect more deeply with people you already know? You can always invite your friends over to learn to make soap. This can be loads of fun, especially if you enjoy teaching, and is a great way to bond as your share your hobby. Beyond that, finding other local soap makers opens up a new avenue for socializing. Organize a soap making meet-up, and start trading tips, tricks, and stories with other soap makers. One fun way to approach this is by hosting a "soap swap" where everyone brings enough of their own soap to share with each other. You walk away with several new soaps to try out, and new friends to share your hobby with. You can also meet soap making friends online, and enjoy trading recipes and photos of your creations. (And, occasionally you may find someone who wants to trade soaps by mail.)

Take Control! My favorite reason for making soap

Taking control! I've had experiences where I fell in love with a product at the store, only to have it discontinued by the manufacturer. When you make your own soap, you pick your favorite recipes, and nobody can ever take those away from you. You also have final control over the ingredients. If you don't want to buy certain oils because you believe that harvesting them is ecologically irresponsible, you don't have to. If you hate lavender, you don't use it. If olive oil irritates your skin, pick another oil. If you're the only person on the planet who likes the smell of chocolate and funnel together, go for it! You get to make all the decisions, and have final control over your soap - it's empowering.

Bathroom Soap Dispenser and Creative SoaspMaking Ideas

A bathroom Soap Dispenser is a product of daily use which can be triggered to give out soap. Soap dispensers come in varied sizes, shapes, styles and colors. It can be mounted on walls, mirrors or on counter tops too. Bathroom soap dispenser's can be either manual or automated. From a dispenser soap generally comes in the form of liquid, powder or foam. Liquid comes under manual dispenser category which is a squeeze plastic bottle that can be disposed off once the liquid soap is finished. Powder used as soap is Borax and it is dispensed through a lever fitted over an metal box containing borax powder. For the soap in foam form, a dual pump dispenser is used which mixes the liquid soap and air together and hence creating lather which is then dispensed out on triggering.

Foam can either be dispensed manually or automatically using the Automated Bathroom Soap Dispenser. It contains motion sensors and is touch free. These are battery powered. When the sensor senses motion under the nozzle it automatically dispenses the soap into the hands user. A automated Dispenser also tells the user whether they have washed their hands properly or not by using an electronic device which keeps track of the time user has washed his hands.

Creative Soap Making Ideas

Soap has nowadays become a very effective gifting accessory too. Some people buy different varieties from the market, wrap them together with attractive wrappings papers or boxes and gift them, while others take a leap forward and make their own soaps and gift them to people on various occasions. Many Creative Soap Making Ideas are there and it can be practiced as hobby or even turn out to be a good employment scheme too.

One Creative Soap Making Idea is to make a soap which has color exactly the same as the color of your bathroom. Use of different miniature soap bits can also help in making multi-colored ones. One can also make a heart shaped one for their loved ones using pink or red color. Who doesn't like a good fragrance? One can make a good smelling soap which can be helpful in rejuvenating after an long, tiring and hectic day at work. You can also make different varieties of it according to the family members in the house and color them according to their favorite colors. For health conscious people, many herbs which are good for health available in the market can be added to soap while making it.

Make Soap at Home - The Soap Making Movement

Soap making is blowing up and becoming more and more mainstream. Everyone wants to learn how to make soap at home. Soon Dove and Caress will be out of business...ok maybe it won't go that far, but who knows. What is up with this new fascination the world has with natural, homemade soap? Why this movement towards learning how to make soap at home?

Nowadays people are demanding to know what's in their products and how safe the ingredients are. Hence this soap making movement. Changing the type of soap you use is the easiest and most convenient way for people to live a more natural and organic lifestyle, because lets face it, everybody uses soap right? Well I should hope so.

Soap is a universal thing, and people are tired of the highly fragranced, drying, worthless crap that we've been using for years. People want to get out of the shower feeling light, refreshed, and moisturized, not like we just walked through the Sahara desert.

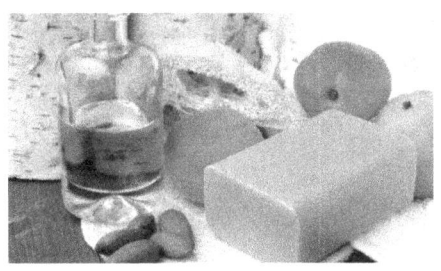

Making soap has many benefits and it's an experience that everyone should have. Making your own soap can have an astonishing effect on the health of your skin. You may notice a new radiance, increased moisture, better elasticity, more even skin tone, and an overall betterment of your skin. Learning how to make soap at home can also have some very good economic benefits also. Initial set up and costs can seem daunting, but in the long run, you will actually save money, and who doesn't want to save money in this economy right now?

And often you will find that making soap is actually really, really fun, and you will find yourself making up new custom recipes, trying a new fragrance, trying a new additive, or even trying your hand at making another beauty product like lotion or bath bombs. You can make soap for women, children, even men. And for children, you can put toys or little surprises in the middle of the soap for them to discover as they use the soap. This is a great motivator to get our children to clean up isn't it?

So there you have it, all the benefits of learning how to make soap at home, and there are a lot more that I didn't mention. So why don't you join the soap making movement?

Aida Kenzie discovered soap making not long ago, and quickly became very passionate about the hobby. She loves learning new things about the art of soap making, and is hoping to meet people from all around the world who are also passionate soap makers, so they can teach her a few tricks of the trade!

Chapter 6: Step By Step Soap Making Process

Now, I've decided that I will be using cold-process as a guide to soap making in this chapter because I find it really helpful especially for those new to soap making who really wants to start right away.

Also, it is because cold process basically starts from scratch, that's why I think it is better to be a starting guide on the soap making process.

Gathering the Ingredients and Tools

For all we know, it is very convenient to have everything you need beforehand because we tend to get organize and therefore the process would be easy and fun, instead of getting troubled because you are panicking since you don't have that particular ingredient in your hand yet and the hardening process is taking place if you stop even for a moment.

By doing this, you'll be able to prevent dangerous situations. Take the time to review all the steps and necessary ingredients I've mentioned so that you can begin!

Soap Making In The Right Place

Of course if you are just beginning to start the process, make sure that all the necessary tools and ingredients must be in a warming area that will help to warm everything up particularly the essential oils on where you basically melt it from the beginning of the process.

Since you have a warm area, you mustn't forget to have a cooling area to harden your finished mixture, and of course because we are literally using the cold process here! Make sure your cooling area must have proper air flow ands ventilation. You can provide coolness by filling up your sink with cold water.

Don't Forget To Measure Your Solid Essential Oils!

After organizing and fixing everything, you must measure your solid oils by means of kitchen scale. You can begin by measuring directly into the pan you are planning to heat your oils in. Of course if possible, you mustn't mix your liquid and solid oils to prevent inconsistency. After you melt the hard oils, get the liquid ones and gradually pour them over all together and start the mixing process.

As for me, I don't really use a lid when heating the hard ingredients, and I heat them on a medium to low fire. If you want to speed up the melting process, break up chunks into pieces.

Creating the Lye

On this process, make sure that you are wearing your gloves and goggles, and of course ensure that your working area is well-ventilated to minimize the vapour of the lye.

When working with lye, make sure that there are no pets, or children around you for the sake of precluding dangerous situations. Of course it would help to minimize the disturbances around you.

Now, measure your lye and water from two separate containers, and for precaution, it is advisable to use a glass container. Take both of the containers into a well-ventilated location and gradually pour the lye into your water and mix using a stainless steel spoon. I've already said it before, but the chemical reaction between water and lye generates great amount of heat so you must always take care.

And here's a great reminder! Never pour your water over the lye because it could cause a mini explosion. Another crucial matter to note is to do all this process in a room temperature ambiance especially for those individuals who are planning to make an herbal soap.

Also, make sure that your water is not lukewarm but a little cold to avoid wild boiling of the mixture. The presence of any kind of sugar is also a taboo for this process.

I've said, cool place, but don't ever put the lye water mixture inside your fridge to prevent unhealthy vapors getting in contact with foods.

Though, working with lye seems a little scary, it is a crucial part of soap making. As I've said, all soap needs lye, including the pre-made soap base use in the melt and pour method.

Be mindful of Temperature

Perhaps one of the most confusing part of making a soap is on what temperature range do you mix your essential oils, and the lye-water solution.

Remember that, the temperature you mix your soap will greatly affect on how your soap will turn out in texture and color. There are various factors that you must consider when picking a soap temperature, and those are type of mold (wood, plastic, or metal), batch size, and what color you are hoping your finished product will become.

If you do the process on a hotter temperature, the color would be more intense. As for me, I usually make soap when my oils are in between 110 and 130 degree F. If you attempt to do the process over 130 degree F, then there's the high possibility of cracking, volcano-ing, and discoloration which you don't really want to happen, right?

The next crucial stuff you must embed in your mind is the lye temperature. Some individuals work with lye mixtures that are in room temperature while their oils are warm. So long as the total temperature of the lye solution and the oils is above the lowest melting point of your essential oils, then everything will most likely turn just fine.

The Trace

This is actually one of the most exciting part of soap making, at least for me. What you want to do first is, pour your lye-water solution through a strainer and get them over your oils. Obviously, the strainer will filter the lye-water solution to get rid of undissolved lye and prevent air bubbles. Next is, submerge the stick mixer into the pan, and tapping it a little to eliminate possible air that might be lurking underneath.

Constantly repeat this process until you come to the so called "Trace". If you don't know, trace is basically the unification of lye-water solution with your oils; ultimately it is also called as saponification. You'll observe that your mixture has reached trace when the consistency is like a thin pudding. Another indicator is when you lift your stick mixer out of the pan and you notice that there are little trails of soap lingering on the surface for a little time.

For tracing, if you don't want to stir for up to three hours, then I don't really recommend using a wisk or spoon. If you want the process to take up to ten minutes, get a stick blender.

Adding Ingredients

After noticing that your mixture had come into trace, you must work fast to add what you want to add especially those delicate ingredients such as antioxidants, herbs, and dried flower petals.

Why add them after the trace? The main reason is that saponification can be super-hot and adding delicate ingredients during that intense phase could destroy their fragrant and beneficial properties.

Another reason is that if you attempt to add whole ingredients such as oats before the trace, then most likely the stick mixer will lift them up too.

Pouring Into The Moulds

Obviously the next process after cooking is pouring the mixture into the moulds.

You have a choice on whether you would like to insulate your soap or not at all. If you insulate your mixture, it will keep the temperature consistent and hot which will ultimately intensify the color and will add a slight transparency to the finished products. This process is also known as the "Gel" state.

You can also insulate your mixture in a wooden box, or just line the top of the soap with a cling film and wrap a large fluffy towel around your moulds. If you decided no to insulate your mixture then its color will be more opaque and lighter.

Regardless if you want to insulate your mixture, you must let it sit for at least a whole day into the mould. This will make the soap to set cool and harden properly. Of course if you attempt to take your soap earlier than planned, then you might be left with a sticky mess.

Cutting Your Finished Product

If you used small bar-sized moulds, then you can just easily pop your soap out of its location and put them on shelves to cure right away. Remember that if you use non-silicone moulds, you might have a hard time of getting the soap out. If this happen to you, you might want to set the finished product into the freezer for around 30 minutes and it will come out automatically with ease.

On the other hand, if you used large moulds, then you can just use any sharp tool to cut your block of soap into bars. If you are a perfectionist and want the loaf of soap to be cut precisely then try getting a professional soap cutter, which are relatively cheap.

Curing Time!

Now your soap seems great! But hey, it's not ready yet since we use the cold process method. What you want to do next is place the sliced bars in a cool, dry, place that has fine ventilation. Don't expose the product to direct sunlight for at least 4 weeks.

If you didn't know, this is now the so-called "curing", and it provides adequate time for your soap to complete saponification process and for all the excess water to evaporate out of the bar. Just don't try to mind your lovely soap, to make the time fast, and before you know it, your soap is now perfectly cured, and ready to use!

Chapter 7: Soap Recipes You Can Make At Home

Oatmeal Cinnamon Exfoliating Bar

Supplies Needed:

1 ½ cup glycerin soap base (clear)

3 tablespoons almond oil

3 tablespoons water

½ cup finely ground oatmeal

½ teaspoon cinnamon powder

Soap mold

Instructions:

Cut glycerin into small cubes.

Put glycerin cubes in a microwave safe glass container and melt for 2-3 minutes in the microwave.

Once the glycerin is melted, allow it to cool for 5 minutes.

Stir in almond oil and water. Add oatmeal and cinnamon and whisk it all together.

Mix until the soap mixture begins to thicken.

Pour the oatmeal cinnamon soap mixture into the mold.

Leave the soap mixture to harden overnight.

Take the soap out of the mold and cut into bars.

Wrap soap in wax paper and store in a cool place, away from direct sunlight.

Lemon Chia Moisturizing Scrub Soap

Supplies Needed:

2 cups soap base (shea butter)

1 cup chia seeds

1 tablespoon lemon essential oil

Soap mold

Instructions:

Spread out half of the chia seeds at the bottom of the soap mold.

Cut the shea butter soap base into cubes.

Put shea butter soap cubes in a microwave safe glass container and melt for around 45 seconds in the microwave. Take the soap base out of the microwave, give it a stir, and put it back into the microwave for a minute until it's completely melted.

Allow the soap base to cool for 5 minutes.

Stir in the lemon essential oil. Add the remaining chia seeds and whisk it all together.

Mix until the soap mixture begins to thicken.

Pour the lemon chia seed soap mixture into the mold.

Leave the soap mixture to cure for at least 24 hours before taking it out of the mold.

Take the soap out of the mold and cut into bars with a sharp knife.

Store soap in wax paper and keep away from direct sunlight.

Vanilla Rose Moisturizing Soap

Supplies Needed:

3 cups soap base (shea butter)

½ cup dried rose petals

1 tablespoon rose essential oil

½ tablespoon vanilla essential oil

Soap mold

Instructions:

Cut shea butter soap base into small chunks and put in a microwave safe glass container.

Melt the shea butter soap base in the microwave in 30 second intervals until you get a liquefied soap.

Set aside the liquefied soap and let it to cool for 5 minutes.

While waiting for the soap to cool, crumble the dried rose petals.

Stir in the rose and vanilla essential oils. Add more if you want the scent to be stronger.

Whisk in the dried rose petals.

Pour the vanilla rose soap mixture into a mold. Allow the soap to dry overnight.

Pop the soap out of the mold and cut into bars before wrapping it in wax paper.

Store soap in a cool dry place, away from direct heat and sunlight.

Sweet Strawberry Soap

Supplies Needed:

2 cups soap base (cocoa butter)

1 cup clear soap base (aloe vera)

1 tablespoon strawberry fragrance oil

1 tablespoon lemon essential oil

¼ teaspoon red mica powder

1 tablespoon distilled water

Soap mold

Instructions:

Cut the cocoa butter soap base into small cubes and put in a heat resistant glass microwaveable bowl.

Heat the cocoa butter soap base in the microwave in 30 second intervals until it's fully melted.

Set aside the liquefied cocoa butter soap base and let it to cool for 5 minutes.

Stir in the strawberry fragrance oil and mix well.

Dissolve the red mica powder in a 1 tablespoon of distilled water before adding it to the cocoa butter soap base. Mix well so you get an even color.

Pour the strawberry cocoa butter soap base into the soap mold. Make sure to only fill it halfway.

Cut the aloe vera soap base into small cubes and put in a heat resistant glass microwaveable bowl.

Heat the aloe vera soap base in the microwave until it's fully melted.

Let it cool for 5 minutes before stirring in the lemon fragrance oil.

Pour the lemon aloe vera soap base into the mold with the strawberry cocoa butter soap base.

1Allow the soap to dry for 24 hours before popping it out of the mold.

1Once hard, slice the soap into bars and wrap it in wax paper.

1Keep away from direct heat and sunlight.

Full Detox Anti Acne Bar

Supplies Needed:

1.5 ounce coconut oil

1.5 ounce cup olive oil

.75 ounce neem oil

.25 ounce castor oil

.75 ounce palm oil

.25 ounce beeswax

.69 ounce lye

1.65 ounce distilled water

20 drops peppermint essential oil

20 drops tea tree essential oil

Soap mold

Instructions:

Carefully pour the lye into the distilled water. Stir gently until the lye is dissolved.

Set aside the lye solution and allow to cool.

Warm the beeswax in a pot on low heat until completely melted. Carefully add the first 5 oils one at a time. Make sure that the oils don't get too hot.

Take the pot off the heat.

Carefully pour the lye and water solution into a pot. Stir all the ingredients together.

Using a hand mixer, blend the soap mixture until you get a creamy pudding consistency.

Put the pot back on low heat and let the soap mixture to cook for about an hour or until the mixture turns transparent.

Stir in the peppermint and tea tree essential oils.

Pour the soap mixture into the soap molds.

Let the soap to cure for 24 hours before cutting them into bars.

1Wrap the soaps in wax paper and store in a cool dry area.

Coconut Milk Moisturizing Soap

Supplies Needed:

4 ounce coconut oil

2 ounce soybean oil

2 ounce extra virgin olive oil

1 ounce shea butter

1 ounce lard

1 ounce castor oil

1.49 ounce lye

3.63 ounce coconut milk

1 tablespoons bentonite clay

Soap mold

Instructions:

Carefully pour the lye into the coconut milk. Stir gently until the lye is dissolved.

Set aside the lye solution and allow to cool.

Mix the first 6 oils together.

Carefully pour the lye and water solution into the oils. Stir all the ingredients together.

Add the bentonite clay.

Using a hand mixer, blend the soap mixture until you get a creamy pudding consistency.

Pour the soap mixture into the soap molds. Let the soap to dry for 24 hours before cutting them into bars.

Wrap the soaps in wax paper and store in a cool dry area for curing.

Activated Charcoal Soap

Supplies Needed:

2 cups soap base (shea butter)

½ cup activated charcoal powder

1 tablespoon tea tree essential oil

1 tablespoon peppermint essential oil

Soap mold

Instructions:

Cut the shea butter soap base into small cubes and heat in the microwave until completely melted. Make sure to use a heat resistant glass container.

Dissolve the activated charcoal powder in 5 tablespoons of melted shea butter soap base.

Pour the charcoal mixture back into the rest of the shea butter soap base.

Stir in the tea tree and peppermint essential oils. Mix well before pouring the soap into the molds.

Cut the soap into bars after allowing the soap to dry for 24 hours.

Wrap in wax paper and store in a cool place.

Skin Brightening Anti-Aging Soap

Supplies Needed:

1 ½ cup soap base (cocoa butter)

2 ½ tablespoons ground rice powder

1 ½ tablespoons distilled water

1 tablespoon lemon essential oil

1 teaspoon vanilla essential oil

Soap mold

Instructions:

Cut cocoa butter soap base into small cubes and place in a glass microwaveable bowl.

Heat the soap base in the microwave in 20 second intervals until it's completely melted.

Allow the cocoa butter soap base to cool for 5 minutes before stirring in the lemon essential oil and vanilla essential oil.

Mix the ground rice powder with the distilled water to make a paste.

Add the rice paste into the soap base and whisk to combine all the ingredients.

Pour the soap into the mold and set aside. Let it harden for 3-4 hours before cutting it into bars.

Wrap soap bars in wax paper and store in a cool dry place.

Rosemary Cooling Soap

Supplies Needed:

2 cups soap base (olive oil)

2 tablespoons loose dried rosemary

2 tablespoons rosemary essential oil

1 tablespoons eucalyptus essential oil

Soap mold

Instructions:

Cut the olive oil soap base into small cubes. Place the cubes in a glass bowl.

Heat the soap base in the microwave in 20 second intervals until completely melted.

Allow the soap base to cool for 5 minutes before stirring in the essential oils.

Add half of the dried rosemary and whisk to mix the ingredients together.

Pour soap into the mold.

Sprinkle the remaining dried rosemary on top of the soap and set aside for 4-5 hours.

Once the soap is hard, remove from the mold and wrap it in wax paper.

Store in a cool dry place, away from direct sunlight.

Lazy Summer Day Soothing Soap

Supplies Needed:

3 cups soap base (goat's milk)

1 tablespoon dried chamomile flowers

2 tablespoons chamomile essential oil

1 tablespoon grapefruit essential oil

1 tablespoon eucalyptus essential oil

Soap mold

Instructions:

Cut goat's milk soap base into small cubes and place in a heat resistant microwave safe bowl.

Heat soap base in the microwave in 20 second intervals until it's completely melted.

Allow soap base to cool for 5 minutes before adding the essential oils.

Whisk the soap mixture until you get a creamy consistency.

Pour the soap mixture into the mold.

Sprinkle the dried chamomile flowers on top of the soap.

Set aside the soap for 4-5 hours to harden.

Cut the soap into bars and wrap it in wax paper. Store it in a cool dry place.

English Garden Cleansing Bar

Supplies Needed:

2 cups soap base (olive oil)

4 tablespoons rose water

2 tablespoons bentonite clay

4 tablespoons jojoba oil

2 tablespoon rose essential essential oil

1 tablespoon lavender essential oil

Soap mold

Instructions:

Cut olive oil soap base into small chunks and melt in a heat resistant microwave safe glass bowl.

Set the microwave to 20 second intervals and heat the soap until it's fully liquefied.

In a separate bowl, mix rose water and bentonite clay until you get a paste.

Allow the melted soap base to cool for 5 minutes before adding the clay paste and essential oils.

Whisk the soap mixture until you get a thick consistency.

Pour the soap mixture into the mold and set it aside.

Let it harden for at least 6 hours before cutting the soap into bars.

Wrap in wax paper. Keep away from direct sunlight.

Morning Coffee Exfoliating Bar

Supplies Needed:

1 ½ cup glycerin soap base (clear)

3 tablespoons olive oil

3 tablespoons water

½ cup unbrewed coffee grounds

1 tablespoon cedarwood essential oil

Soap mold

Instructions:

Cut glycerin into small cubes.

Put glycerin cubes in a microwave safe glass container and melt for 2-3 minutes in the microwave.

Once the glycerin is melted, allow it to cool for 5 minutes.

Stir in olive oil and water. Add coffee grounds and cedarwood essential oil and whisk it all together.

Mix until the soap mixture begins to thicken.

Pour the coffee soap mixture into the mold.

Leave the soap mixture to harden overnight.

Take the soap out of the mold and cut into bars.

Wrap soap in wax paper and store in a cool place, away from direct sunlight.

Chocolate Mint Exfoliating Bar

Supplies Needed:

2 cups soap base (shea butter)

½ cup cocoa powder

1 tablespoon peppermint essential oil

1 tablespoon dried mint

Soap mold

Instructions:

Spread out half of the cocoa powder at the bottom of the soap mold.

Cut the shea butter soap base into cubes.

Put shea butter soap cubes in a microwave safe glass container and melt for around 45 seconds in the microwave. Take the soap base out of the microwave, give it a stir, and put it back into the microwave for a minute until it's completely melted.

Allow the soap base to cool for 5 minutes.

Stir in the peppermint essential oil. Add the remaining cocoa powder and dried mint and whisk all the ingredients together.

Mix until the soap mixture begins to thicken.

Pour the chocolate mint soap mixture into the mold.

Leave the soap mixture to cure for at least 24 hours before taking it out of the mold.

Take the soap out of the mold and cut into bars with a sharp knife.

Store soap in wax paper and keep away from direct sunlight.

Lavender Fields Moisturizing Soap

Supplies Needed:

3 cups soap base (shea butter)

½ cup dried lavender flowers

2 tablespoons lavender essential oil

1 tablespoon peppermint essential oil

Soap mold

Instructions:

Cut shea butter soap base into small chunks and put in a microwave safe glass container.

Melt the shea butter soap base in the microwave in 30 second intervals until you get a liquefied soap.

Set aside the liquefied soap and let it to cool for 5 minutes.

While waiting for the soap to cool, crumble the dried lavender flowers.

Stir in lavender and peppermint essential oils. Add more if you want the scent to be stronger.

Whisk in the dried lavender flowers.

Pour the lavender soap mixture into a mold. Allow the soap to dry and harden overnight.

Pop the soap out of the mold and cut into bars.

Wrap soap bars in wax paper and store in a cool dry place, away from direct heat and sunlight.

Oasis Dreams Moisturizing Soap

Supplies Needed:

3 cups soap base (cocoa butter)

1 tablespoon sandalwood essential oil

½ tablespoon lemon essential oil

½ tablespoon rosehip essential oil

¼ teaspoon blue mica powder

1 tablespoon distilled water

Soap mold

Instructions:

Cut the cocoa butter soap base into small cubes and put in a heat-safe glass microwaveable bowl.

Heat the cocoa butter soap base in the microwave in 30 second intervals until it's fully melted.

Set aside the liquefied cocoa butter soap base and let it to cool for 5 minutes.

Stir in all the essential oils and mix well.

Dissolve the blue mica powder in 1 tablespoon of distilled water before adding it to the cocoa butter soap base. Mix well until you get an even color.

Pour the soap into the mold.

Allow the soap to cure for 24 hours before popping it out of the mold.

Slice the soap into bars and wrap it in wax paper.

Keep away from direct heat and sunlight.

Floral Clear Skin Soap

Supplies Needed:

1.25 ounce extra virgin olive oil

1.5 ounce neem oil

.75 palm oil

.25 ounce jojoba oil

.35 ounce emu oil

.25 ounce beeswax

.71 ounce lye

1.85 ounce distilled water

20 drops lavender essential oil

20 drops rose essential oil

Soap mold

Instructions:

Carefully pour the lye into the distilled water. Stir gently until the lye is dissolved.

Set aside the lye solution and allow to cool.

Warm the beeswax in a pot on low heat until completely melted. Carefully add the first 5 oils one at a time. Make sure that the oils don't get too hot.

Take the pot off the heat.

Carefully pour the lye and water solution into a pot. Stir all the ingredients together.

Using a hand mixer, blend the soap mixture until you get a creamy pudding consistency.

Put the pot back on low heat and let the soap mixture to cook for about an hour or until the mixture turns transparent.

Stir in the lavender and rose essential oils.

Pour the soap mixture into the soap molds. Let the soap to cure for 24 hours before cutting them into bars.

Wrap the soaps in wax paper and store in a cool dry area.

Cool And Refreshing Anti Spot Soap

Supplies Needed:

2 cups soap base (aloe vera)

1 teaspoon dried mint leaves

½ teaspoon tea tree essential oil

½ teaspoon lavender essential oil

½ teaspoon lemon essential oil

Soap mold

Instructions:

Cut the aloe vera soap base into small cubes and heat in the microwave until completely melted. Make sure to use a heat-safe glass container.

Allow the soap base to cool for 5 minutes before adding the dried mint leaves.

Stir in the tea tree, lavender, and lemon essential oils. Mix well before pouring the soap into the molds.

Cut the soap into bars after letting it harden and dry for 24 hours.

Wrap in wax paper and store in a cool place.

Almond Milk Anti-Aging Soap

Supplies Needed:

1 ½ cup soap base (goat's milk)

2 ½ tablespoons bentonite clay

2 tablespoons distilled water

2 tablespoons almond essential oil

1 tablespoon vanilla essential oil

Soap mold

Instructions:

Cut goat's milk soap base into small cubes and place in a glass microwaveable bowl.

Heat the soap base in the microwave in 20 second intervals until it's completely melted.

Allow the goat's milk soap base to cool for 5 minutes before stirring in the almond oil and vanilla essential oil.

Mix the bentonite clay with the distilled water to make a paste.

Add the clay paste into the soap base and whisk to combine all the ingredients.

Pour the soap into the mold and set aside. Let it harden for at least 6 hours before cutting it into bars.

Wrap soap bars in wax paper and store in a cool dry place.

La Vie En Rose Nourishing Bar

Supplies Needed:

2 cups soap base (olive oil)

1 tablespoon loose dried rose petals

2 tablespoons rose essential oil

1 tablespoon rosehip essential oil

Soap mold

Instructions:

Cut the olive oil soap base into small cubes. Place the cubes in a glass bowl.

Heat the soap base in the microwave in 20 second intervals until completely melted.

Allow the soap base to cool for 5 minutes before stirring in the essential oils.

Add half of the dried rose petals and whisk to mix the ingredients together.

Pour soap into the mold.

Sprinkle the remaining dried rose petals on top of the soap and set aside for 4-5 hours.

Once the soap is hard, remove from the mold wrap it in wax paper.

Store in a cool dry place, away from direct sunlight.

Spring Blooms Nourishing Bar

Supplies Needed:

3 cups soap base (aloe vera)

1 tablespoon dried lavender flowers

2 tablespoons geranium essential oil

1 tablespoon lavender essential oil

1 tablespoon lemongrass essential oil

Soap mold

Instructions:

Cut aloe vera soap base into small cubes and place in a heat resistant microwave safe bowl.

Heat soap base in the microwave in 20 second intervals until it's melted.

Allow soap base to cool for 5 minutes before adding the essential oils.

Whisk the soap mixture until you get a creamy consistency.

Pour the soap mixture into the mold.

Sprinkle the dried lavender flowers on top of the soap.

Set aside the soap for 4-5 hours to harden.

Cut the soap into bars and wrap it in wax paper. Store it in a cool dry place.

Chapter 8: Soap-Making Methods

There are many ways to make soap. I'll bet that you didn't realize how many forms of soap making there actually are! When talking about bars soaps alone there are so many types, it boggles the mind. Cold process, hot process, melt and pour, rebatchingsoap. Those are the basic types of soap that I will describe in detail.

Melt and Pour Soap: Technically, all handmade soaps are Glycerin Soaps." In many commercial soaps, all the extra glycerin is harvested out. Thus, all handmade soaps are glycerin rich.

In today's market, the term "Glycerin Soap" is commonly used to refer to clear soap. Generally, the clear soap has extra glycerin added to it.

Clear soap base can be purchased in large blocks to be melted down, colored or placed into molds. This type of soap is called "Melt and Pour" and the artistry of melt and pour is called Soap Casting. Melt and Pour soap making is gaining in popularity because of its ease of use. There are no significant safety measures. Even Children can do it. It's a great outlet for creative types of personalities.

is really straightforward. All you have to do is to:

buy a pre-made soap base

 Melt the soap base into a liquid, add extra ingredients like soap dye, essential oils, herbs and nutrients

Pour the soap into your mold of choice

Decorate and design if desired

Let it harden.

Although this could potentially be the easiest of all the soap making methods, it is a wonderful way for beginners to start making their own soap.

Cold Process Method: This is by far the most traditional method of soap making. The process involves combining fats or oils with lye and water. Unlike melt and pour soap making, the cold process method involves creating your own soap base from scratch. Through a chemical reaction called saponification. During saponification, the oils and lye mix and become soap – the process takes approximately six weeks to fully complete.

The amount of fats and lye must be estimated using a saponification chart. The measurements must be exact so that there is no extra hydroxide.

Historically, lye used in the cold process was made from scratch using rainwater and ashes. Soapmakers deemed the lye solution ready for use when an egg would float in it. Homemade lye making for this process was unpredictable and therefore eventually led to the discovery of the sodium hydroxide

Cold process soap making requires the use of lye and the use of safety equipment, such as goggles and gloves. Cold process soap is known for its hard and long lasting quality.

Hot Process Soaps: Hot processing is usually used to create liquid soaps. The hot process soap making method is very similar to the cold process method except that heat is used to speed up the saponification process. The simple explanation is that you take all your ingredients, and add them to a pot that is then placed over a heat source. Heat is applied at different stages using an oven, crock pot, or even a microwave, depending on your method.

One huge disadvantage to this style of soap making is that it can sometimes be difficult to remove the soap from its mold. Also, depending on your hot process method, it can sometimes be hard to get the soap into the mold. Hot process soap making has a huge advantage in that the cure time is greatly reduced. So, you will not have to wait for weeks to use your new soap!

Chapter 9: Hot Processed Soaps

Coffee Antioxidant Soap

Ingredients:

- 24 ounces of olive oil

- 32 ounces of coconut oil

- 4 ounces of castor oil

- 1 ounce of jojoba oil or cocoa butter

- 260 grams of lye crystals

- 20 ounces of coffee, brewed or triple strength, cooled (the water used for the coffee should be distilled water)

- 60 ml of cinnamon oil

- 60 ml of lemon or sweet orange oil

- 90 grams of ground dry coffee

- 15 grams of cinnamon, ground

- 15 grams of cloves, ground

- 15 grams of dried ginger or ginseng, ground

Directions:

Make a lye and coffee solution. Add the lye to the coffee and stir. Let it cool to room temperature or not more than 40 degrees centigrade.

Mix your oils, except for the cocoa butter and cool the mixture.

Mix the oil and the lye solution in a deep pot. Blend until the mixture creates a trace.

Add the ground coffee and the other ground powders. Give it a quick mix using the hand mixer.

Place the pot onto the double boiler. Cook over low heat for at least an hour. Stir occasionally in the first 30 minutes.

Check every 15 minutes to see if a trace appears.

Meanwhile, melt the cocoa butter and let it cool.

After an hour, give your oil a stir. Draw a line across your mixture. If the line takes two to five seconds to disappear, it's ready

Turn off the heat. Add the cocoa butter and the essential oils. Mix thoroughly.

Pour into your mold, lined with wax paper or butcher paper.

Let the soap stand for 24 hours before slicing.

*The soap can be used immediately. But, if you want the soap to not melt easily, you may cure it in open air for 2 to 6 weeks.

Avocado And Mango Swirl Soap

Ingredients:

- 400 grams of coconut oil

- 155 grams of palm oil
- 36 grams of Shea butter
- 36 grams of avocado butter
- 69 grams of avocado oil
- 120 grams of lye
- 231 ml of distilled water
- 30 ml of mango fragrance oil
- Calendula petals or dried flower petals (optional)
- ¼ teaspoon green mica powder
- ¼ teaspoon yellow mica powder

Directions:

Make the lye solution. Let it cool down.

Melt your oils and mix them well. Let it cool down.

When the oil and the lye solution has a temperature below 40 degrees centigrade, add the lye solution to the oil and mix with a hand mixer.

When a light trace appears, stop mixing. Place the pot over a double boiler. Stir the mixture occasionally during the first 30 minutes. Check every 15 minutes to see if the mixture develops a trace.

When the mixture begins to trace, add the extracts.

Divide the mixture into three parts. Add the yellow mica powder to one part and mix. Add the green mica to the other part and mix. Return the colored parts to the plain part and mix lightly or until the colors form a marble swirl in the plain mixture.

Add the dried petals, if using. Mix.

Pour into the mold lined with butcher paper. Let it stand for 24 hours before slicing.

Chapter 10: Homemade Soap For Exfoliation

For this soap, you need; one pound of goat's milk, glycerin soap and a Melton pour soap base, one tablespoon of coconut oil, and a four tablespoon of poppy seeds. You also need one mold; you can use any mold you find in the craft store in the soap making aisle.

STEP 1

To start off, you need one pound of soap base, so that's going to be roughly half of the soap base; it's on a two-pound box, you cut the soap in half, and then you cut each individual cube in half and fill it and put it into a liquid measuring cup, pop it in the microwave for a minute or two. Let it meltdown and then add the remaining cubes. Once you're done, make sure that you stir thoroughly and that everything is melted, and all the chunks, even at the bottom, have been melted.

STEP 2

Next, you're going to take that coconut oil, and you'll need a tablespoon. Instead of adding it directly to soap, you heat it up. It only takes about 30 seconds or less in the microwave, so watch it. Once it's in liquid form, you're going to add that to your soap. Ensure you stir it well so that it spreads evenly throughout your base.

STEP 3

Also, you need a four tablespoon of poppy seeds, a four tablespoon might not seem like a lot, but it's going to be just plenty for this recipe. Once you pour it in, make sure you stir really well. You want it to spread evenly. The good news from the goat's milk is that it's actually created with the suspension formula, which means that the poppy seeds won't sink to the bottom. They will flow evenly throughout your soap once it's molded. So once you're ready, just start pouring into your heart-shaped molds. This recipe for one pound usually yields six bars of soap. And once it's in the mold, you are to let it sit for a couple of hours. Sometimes it's done in 40 minutes, but sometimes you should allow it to rest overnight. You just want to make sure that they're not warm at all. And then once you're done, pop it out, and your yield is a beautiful gorgeous heart-shaped soap that your customers would love to have as a gift or just a way to treat themselves. It's a perfect exfoliator using the poppy seeds. The goat's milk and coconut oil are perfect for the skin.

How to Make a Soap for Skin Tan

Ingredients you will need include; five soap bases and a transparent soap base. These are easy to use and save you from handling caustic soda. Please make sure you get one, which is sulfate-free; they are easily available online.

You can use any clay such as bentonite clay, dense clay, or even Multani. It unlocks the skin force, controls oil formation, gently exfoliates, adds glow. It makes the skin softer too.

Go to any beauty store to get poppy seeds, it acts as a natural exfoliator, and it's super gentle on the skin due to its fine ground granules.

Papaya essential oil imparts some glow when used. You can use a lavender rose or peppermint essential oil to restore, calm, and soothe sun-damaged skin.

Liquid food color to give the soap beautiful color.

Rubbing alcohol, also known as isopropanol alcohol. It is required to fuse layers and give the soap a neater finish, and to remove the bubbles.

The pretty mold, to give a beautiful shape to your soap, and some microwave-safe containers.

Step 1

When making soap of two sides, both having the respective benefits, where one side will act as a gentle scrubber having poppy seeds, and the other side will provide softening as it will have to make the exfoliating side. The first step is to take a microwave-safe container. You need to cut the transparent soap base into small chunks and melt it in the microwave, giving it 30 seconds heat per minute.

Step 2

Once it is melted, you are going to add a few drops of orange food color. About eight drops of papaya essential oil and a teaspoon full of poppy seeds. Mix them all and pour the shea butter to the mold only halfway.

Step 3

Spray rubbing alcohol to remove any bubbles, let it sit for some time until the layer thickens. Now, moving on to the next side, the soft one, take another container and melt some white soap base following the same process as mentioned before.

Step 4

Once it has melted, you need to add one teaspoon of the clay and a few drops of papaya essential oil. Mix them all. Now take the exfoliating soap mold and check if it is set, then go ahead and spray some rubbing alcohol over it. Pour the hot substitution that we need carefully over the crappy mold. And let it sit for a couple of hours in the mold, and you have a two-sided soap ready.

Homemade Soap for the Winter

This soap is super moisturizing and hydrating. It makes the skin soft, glowing, and radiant.

Step 1

Get your aloe vera soap base, get your Multani Mutti, it is great for cleansing the skin and removing excess oil and light ache pimples.

Get your sandalwood powder; it is suitable for cleansing the skin and making it glowing and radiant.

Glycerin is a great moisturizer, and it retains water in the skin.

Olive oil is an anti-aging agent and improves the health of the skin.

Vitamin C and vitamin E capsules are essential components for healthy skin.

Rose is an anti-bacterial and antioxidants.

Step 2

Start with cutting the soap base into small pieces, microwave it for about 1-2 minutes, then grind it in the mixer grinder and make a powder. Start mixing all the ingredients, 3 tablespoons of glycerin, then mix it. Add 2 tablespoons of Multani Mutti and sandalwood powder 2 tablespoons, continue mixing it.

Step 3

Add your rose petals to it; you can also use dried rose petals, set your mold, and press the mixture into the mold to take the shape of your mold without leaving space. After that, you place it in the refrigerator for about 10-15 minutes, and your soap is ready.

Homemade Soap for Dry Skin

Step 1

Cut 1 bar of soap base into chunks and place it in a large microwave-safe container. For 30 seconds, microwave and stir, then microwave in 10 seconds intervals stirring it periodically, until soap is melted.

Step 2

If you don't have a container large enough for all the soap at once, you can melt it down in batches and transfer the melted soap to a larger non-microwave-safe bowl.

Step 3

Allow the soap to cool slightly until a "skin" is formed on top, add 2 teaspoons of honey and 3 drops of essential oil (optional) and stir.

Step 4

Add ¼ cup of lightly grounded oatmeal and stir until it sinks. If the soap is still too hot, wait for it to cool more then stir again. Spray mold with rubbing alcohol. This is optional but helpful. Then pour the soap into the mold, spray it with rubbing alcohol and allow it to cool overnight.

It doesn't need additional cure time; it is ready for use.

Chapter 11: Easy Techniques For Newbies

Simple cleanser making can regularly appear to be incomprehensible. Numerous formulas require forms that incorporate burning lye and hours of blending notwithstanding sitting tight for the soap to cure for about six weeks. At the point when attempting to discover simple soap making formulas, it might give the idea that simple cleanser making is anything besides simple.

The techniques for frosty and hot procedure cleaner making require the planning of a soap base. This requires a lie blend and the frequently tedious and possibly risky procedure of consolidating the lye mixture with dissolved oils.

The simple pour and form technique for cleanser making spares you the progressions of making the cleaner base. There are pre-made soap bases in numerous plans that make the shampoo making the process as essential as liquefying the base, including hues and aroma and filling a mold.

At the point when the solvent is cooled you require just expel the cleanser from the mold and your simple soap making undertaking is finished. Soap making packs that contain every one of the fixings to make a particular kind of soap are additionally accessible. The accompanying is a great formula for pour and shape soap. It produces proficient showing up results and is unquestionably simple soap making taking care of business.

BERRY Simple BAR Cleanser BARIngredients:

* Murky white cleanser base

* Clear shampoo base

* Vanilla, raspberry, and blueberry scent oils

* Dropper for shading and fragrance oils

* Restorative colorants. Purple, blue and lilac (utilize an infinitesimal measure of purple to accomplish a lilac shading)

* Cooking splash for mere arrival of cleanser from the mold

* Rubbing liquor utilized for air pocket decrease

* 4 plastic compartments and one roll formed cleanser mold

Directions:

1. Start with a white secret base, dissolve the base and empty ¾ glasses base into each of the three separate plastic holders. Soap molds can likewise be utilized.

2. Add shading to every bunch with a dropper. Shift the shade of every band.

Add shading in little adds up to acquire fancied impact. Keep in mind that all the more shading can be added to obtain the sought result however shading can't be expelled.

3. Permit the cleanser to solidify. As the solvent thickens, splash the roll formed soap mold with cooking shower and evacuate any abundance oil with paper toweling.

4. At the point when the three separate groups are cooled and solidified, leave and cut into various estimated vast pieces.

5. Fill the chunk mold with the cleanser pieces, utilizing pieces from every cluster to change the situation of the distinctive hue clumps.

6. Keep on filling the frame to 2/3 full. At the point when the mold is 1/3 full shower the cleanser pieces with liquor to forestall gurgling. Rehash when 2/3 full.

7. Melt the clear cleaner base and fill a 2-container measuring glass. Empty this blend into a plastic compartment.

8. Include the scent: Utilize sparingly and include more for more prominent aroma content: 2 Sections vanilla 1 Section raspberry 1 Section blueberry.

9. As the blend, cools evacuate skin with a spoon and pour the mixture over the cleanser pieces in the mold. Pour gradually until the mold is filled. Utilize the liquor to wipe out rises at first glance.

10. Permit the mold to solidify for four hours or until totally cooled.

11. At the point when the cleanser has calmed totally expel the cleanser from the mold, and cut.

Proficient is looking excellent and straightforward to make cleaner! Congrats!

Chapter 12: Hot Process Soap Making

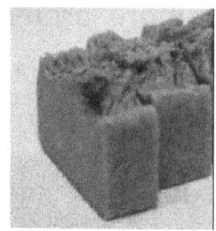

"Hot" soap from scratch is interesting due to the fact that it can be enriched with all sorts of useful additives, and can already be used the next day after making.

To make soap by hot method, you must first act on the script of cold soap process and when it reaches the "trace" stage, put it to cook.

You can make soap by the hot method in the following ways:

• over water bath;

- in the oven.

Each option has its own little features. It's up to you to decide which option is more preferable.

Advantages of making soap over the water bath: the whole process of soap making is constantly in front of your eyes, and if necessary, you can adjust it quickly; mixing soap mass is somewhat simpler and eliminates the possibility of getting burnt while taking the pan out of the oven. Advantages of making soap in the oven: the soap mass is heated evenly and the soaping process is faster; it takes less time for the soap to be mixed; In my opinion, this method is perfect for those who can have the oven temperature precisely controlled.

How long does it take to make soap?

Making soap by hot method usually takes from 2 to 4 hours. In an oven, this process is faster, since soap mass is heated more evenly. For the soap is made over the water bath faster, you need to monitor the level of water in the bottom of the pan: it should be equal to the soap mass level.

Soap is ready when soaping reaction between fats and alkaline solution is completed. And it proceeds faster when oil and alkaline solution are mixed with blender.

> How do I know that the mass is well stirred?
>
> The soap consistency mass will prompt us about this, i.e. "trace". Thick "trace" indicates that everything is well mixed and the soaping reaction has started.
>
> In the process of blender mixing oils break into small droplets, which are distributed in alkaline solution. An emulsion is formed and the stable it is, the faster the soaping reaction will be.

The temperature is also vital for the rate of soaping reaction. After mixing the soap mass you need to put it warm up. At this stage, when the temperature rises to 80 ° C, a rapid soaping occurs of about 80% fat, and this process takes approximately an hour. Further, the temperature is maintained at 95-105 ° C for several hours (2-4). The reaction at this stage is slow since alkali concentration decreased and the concentration of glycerol increases. It is the "gel" stage- soap becomes translucent, like jelly. After completing the soaping process the mass becomes wax like consistency and checking the pH with the help of indicator paper provides an indication of 7-8.

About test strips ...

The strips for measuring the acidity (pH) have a scale from 0 to 12 (or 14):

- 0 corresponds to a highly acidic environment;

- 5.5 - slightly acidic environment: corresponds to the average acidity of human skin;

- 7.0 - neutral level (distilled water has this level);

- 12 - strong alkaline environment.

Using pH-strips for home soap making must be adjusted for the fact that they were created only in order to determine what environment we have: acidic or alkaline, and not to show the exact level. For this reason, the acidity of soap is equal to 7-8 on the test paper, should not be taken as the correct value, but only as a signal that the soap is ready.

Raw soap has high alkali content. While soap maturation it decreases and the pH of the ready soap is 8-10.

As you can see, the test strips have a large measurement error. To obtain accurate data it is necessary to use a special pH-meter. Many try the soap readiness on the tongue: if it does not sting, then it is ready.

How to measure the pH in soap?

This can be done using a special test paper. Just dip one end of the strip into the liquid soap mass for a few seconds, remove and compare the resulting color with the reference scale. If soap is cooked and firm, then you need it lightly moistened with water, foamed, and dip the strip into the ready soap solution.

Raw soap will dye yellow litmus strip in navy blue color, and ready soap - green or blue-green.

So, for you to visualize the soap making process by hot method, I can suggest you a small workshop.

1. Weigh fluid (ice) for alkaline solution

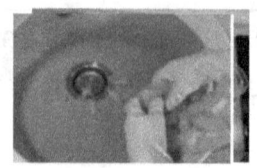

2. Weigh the solid and liquid oils separately

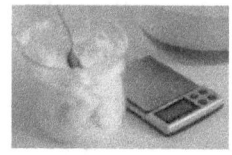

3. Weigh alkali

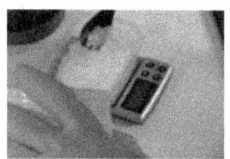

4. Fill sink with ice-water for cooling

5. Gently stir alkali into the glass with ice (water)

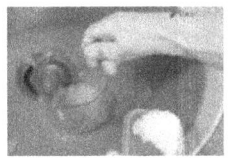

6. Melt solid oils over a water bath

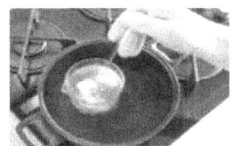

7. Measure the temperature of the alkaline solution and oils

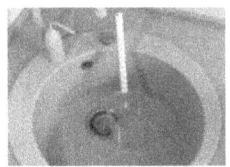

8. Combine the solid and liquid oils

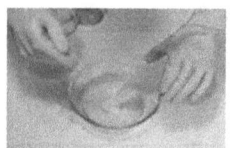

9. Pour oil alkaline solution through a sieve

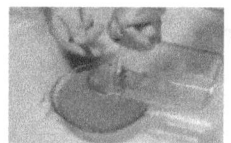

10. Begin stirring it with a blender

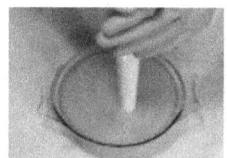

So far the process has been similar to the cold method. Further comes the actual process of soap making.

11. Turn the blender and bring it up to the "trace" stage

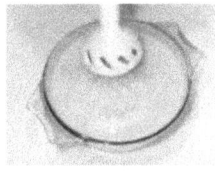

12. Cover the saucepan with lid

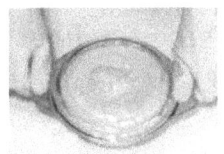

13. Put over a water bath or oven to cook

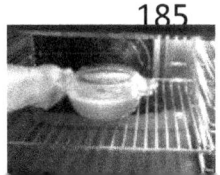

14. After 15-30 minutes the soap becomes gelatinous (gel)

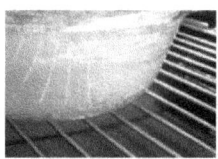

15. If necessary, stir the soap mass

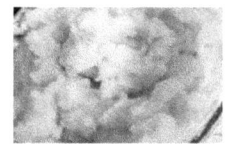

As you already understood, when making soap by a hot method it gradually changes from a gel state to a wax-like. On the surface of the soap, crust may be formed, so it should be mixed as needed (once every 40-60 minutes).

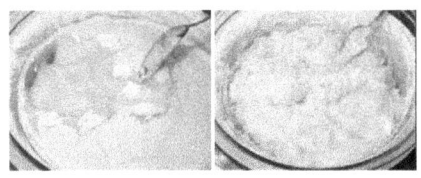

As the soap is being made, get ready for the final stage: weigh oils for superfat, measure useful additives, cover the mold for soap with parchment, tracing paper or other grease repellent paper.

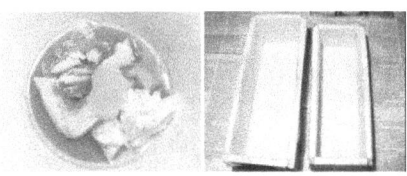

Once you have determined that the soap is ready, utility is added, superfat, essential oils and it is decomposed into special molds.

16. Add the utility (e.g, banana puree)

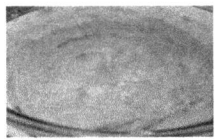

17. Add superfat and essential oils

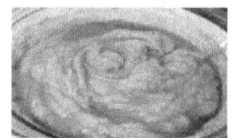

18. Transfer it into the mold and knock well with fingers

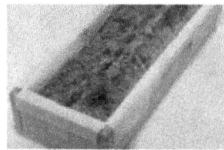

19. After 12-24 hours, remove from the mold

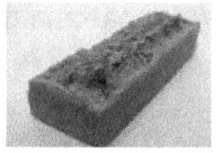

20. Cut the soap into pieces

So you can use this soap the next day. If you let the soap dry for a few days, the excess moisture evaporates and soap will only get better.

Conclusion

Soap making is not really a hard activity even if it involves some seemingly-complicated ingredients and stuffs. In fact, gathering and using those ingredients in your soap making process is one of the most fun and exciting part of crafting your very own soap especially because you can make use of them for possible soap making experiments.

Well, of course the ingredients involved in your recipes are only fragments of the real fun. Perhaps the most delightful part of soap making (atleast in my own opinion) is when you are patiently waiting for the soap to completely hardened and are getting excited of taking it inside the bathroom.

How about you? Perhaps you haven't still discovered the cozy yet fun feeling of making soap. If that's the case, why not start making your very own soap now? I tell you, it's super easy, fun, frugal, and absolutely delighting!

www.ingramcontent.com/pod-product-compliance
Lightning Source LLC
Chambersburg PA
CBHW071830080526
44589CB00012B/971